W0111280

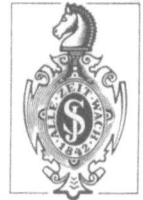

J. C. Frauenthal

Mathematical Modeling
in Epidemiology

Springer-Verlag
Berlin Heidelberg New York 1980

James C. Frauenthal
Department of Applied Mathematics and Statistics
State University of New York
Stony Brook, N.Y. 11794/USA

ISBN-13: 978-3-540-10328-8   e-ISBN-13: 978-3-642-67795-3
DOI: 10.1007/978-3-642-67795-3

Library of Congress Cataloging in Publication Data. Frauenthal, J. C. 1944-.
Mathematical modeling in epidemiology. (Universitext). Bibliography: p.
Includes index. 1. Epidemiology-Mathematical models. 2. Mathematical models.
I. Title.
RA652.2.M3F72. 614.4'0724. 80-21231

© by Springer-Verlag Berlin Heidelberg 1980

2141/3140-543210

Preface

The text of this book is derived from courses taught by the author in the Department of Applied Mathematics and Statistics at the State University of New York at Stony Brook. The audience for these courses was composed almost entirely of fourth year undergraduate students majoring in the mathematical sciences. The students had ordinarily completed four semesters of calculus and one of probability. Few had any prior experience with differential equations, stochastic processes, or epidemiology. It also seems prudent to mention that the author's background is in engineering and applied mathematics and not in epidemiology; it is hoped that this is not painfully obvious.

The topics covered in this book have in some cases been modified from the way they were originally presented. However, care has been taken to include a suitable amount of material for a one semester course; the temptation to add gratuitous subject matter has been resisted. Similarly, when a choice between clarity and rigor was available, the more easily understood exposition was selected.

By looking only at the table of contents, the casual reader could be easily misled into thinking that the main concern of this book is with epidemiology. This is not the case. The purpose of this book is to illustrate the process of formulating and solving mathematical models. Epidemiology is employed as a pedagogic device to provide unity and intuitive appeal to the various mathematical ideas discussed; when the epidemiological terminology is stripped away, what remains is a collection of deterministic and stochastic mathematical models.

The topics ciscussed in this book fall quite naturally into two groups. The first contains general models for the spread of a disease (or rumor or altered state) through a susceptible population. Different ways of keeping track of the state of the population are considered by using different treatments of time and numbers. In Chapter 1 (Deterministic Epidemic Models), three deterministic mathematical models for an epidemic outbreak of a contagious disease are developed. Each successive model attempts to rectify the faults of the prior formulations. The final model is interesting in that it leads to the conclusion that there is a disease threshold or minimum number of susceptibles needed for the occurrence of an epidemic, a condition not intentionally built in to the mathematics. The second chapter (Rumors and Mousetraps) attempts to illustrate the distinction between a deterministic and a stochastic formulation of two epidemic-like processes. The models are first posed in deterministic terms; in each case it is soon apparent that more than one possible outcome can occur. To avoid the necessity of introducing probability densities, the expected evolution of the system is calculated. In Chapter 3 (Stochastic Epidemic Models), the models of Chapter 1 are re-derived in full stochastic form. It is discovered that the probabilistic versions are considerably harder to solve than their deterministic analogues, and that they lead to somewhat different results. Chapter 4 (Chain Binomial Models) investigates both the deterministic and stochastic versions of a model for an epidemic outbreak within a small population. The model is strongly reminiscent of the ones discussed in Chapter 2. However, the stochastic model employed conditions the present state of the system on prior states. Several methods are discussed for deconditioning the probabilities, and the outcome of the stochastic and deterministic versions are compared. Chapter 5 (Branching Process Model) investigates the application of the well-known Galton-Watson branching process to a small epidemic within a large population of susceptibles.

The second portion of the book is concerned with models for specific diseases. These have been included to allow a careful discussion of modeling only the salient points of a larger problem. Chapter 6 (Smallpox Vaccination Discontinuation) studies the question: given a rare disease for which there is a vaccine, when does it become better to risk the consequences of an epidemic than to incur the mortality associated with the vaccine? The optimal solution is found by investigating various stages of an outbreak using stochastic models. In Chapter 7 (Schistosomiasis Eradication) a mathematical model is constructed to explain a qualitative observation about schistosomiasis, a host-vector disease in which humans are the hosts and snails are the vectors. By identifying the critical phase in the disease process (which occurs in the humans' circulatory systems), a specialized model turns out to be sufficient to explain the paradox. Chapter 8 (Gonorrhea) looks at another troublesome situation: the recent rise in the number of cases of gonorrhea within the United States. The model is used to show that we are not in fact experiencing the beginning of an epidemic. The final chapter (Sickle Cell Anemia) looks at an explanation for the occurrence of a well-known genetic disease by means of models from Mendelian genetics. It is hoped that students will develop enthusiasm for mathematical applications based upon seeing situations which they understand treated with fairly sophisticated techniques.

At the end of each chapter a number of problems have been included to provide practice with mathematical concepts and techniques. Solutions will be found at the end of the book. It is suggested that during a one semester course all problems be solved by students. Without this level of activity the mathematical details cannot be adequately appreciated. Also at the end of each chapter is an annotated list of references.

Most of the ideas and models contained in this book are not original, and to their creators I owe a debt of gratitude. I would like to express my thanks in particular to Norman T.J. Bailey, Chief of the Health Statistical Methodology Section of the World Health Organization and more than anyone else the guiding force in mathematical epidemiology. I should also like to express my sincere appreciation to the Alfred P. Sloan Foundation, whose support greatly facilitated the preparation of this book.

Stony Brook, New York James C. Frauenthal
April 1980

Table of Contents

Chapter 1. Deterministic Epidemic Models

We begin by looking at a sequence of three increasingly complicated mathematical models for the development of an epidemic of a contagious disease. The first model is so simple as to be almost entirely unrealistic; however, its shortcomings suggest how it can be improved. The second model, which results from modifying the first model, is considerably better, but still leads to unacceptable results. The third model is likewise an outgrowth of the previous models. Although still imperfect, the third model manifests a property which was not built into the formulation explicitly, but which is in fact observable in an actual epidemic of a contagious disease.

Before looking at specific models, we will make a number of assumptions which will be common to all of the models:

   a.   The disease is transmitted by contact between an
        infected individual and a susceptible individual.

   b.   There is no latent period for the disease, hence
        the disease is transmitted instantaneously upon
        contact.

   c.   All susceptible individuals are equally susceptible
        and all infected individuals are equally infectious.

   d.   The population under consideration is fixed in size.
        This means that no births or migration occurs, and
        all deaths are taken into account.

I. The Trivial Model

Consider a population which is effectively infinite in size. Initially everyone in the population is susceptible to a contagious disease, with the exception of a small number of individuals who are already infected.

Let the independent variable be time, t, and also let:

I(t) = number of infected individuals at time t

B = average number of contacts with susceptible
individuals which lead to a new infective per
unit time per infective in the population.

It is a simple matter to deduce the number of infected individuals at time t+Δt in terms of the number of infectives at time t. Clearly, I(t+Δt) is just the sum of the number of infectives at time t, I(t), plus the number of new infectives who contract the disease in the time interval from t to t+Δt. In mathematical notation,

$$I(t+\Delta t) = I(t) + B\,I(t)\,\Delta t$$

n.b. It should be clear that we have already encountered a small
inconsistency. In general, one would not expect I(t+Δt) to be an
integer even if I(t) was an integer. Instead of trying to cope
with this problem, we will recognize that our model is inexact,
and will interpret I(t) to the nearest integer. Since we will
discover that the number of infectives grows without bound, this
imprecision will not be serious.

Next, rearrange the equation into the form:

$$\frac{I(t+\Delta t) - I(t)}{\Delta t} = B\,I(t)$$

and then let $\Delta t \to 0$. This yields

$$\frac{dI(t)}{dt} = B\,I(t)$$

We recognize this as a simple ordinary differential equation. By virtue of its form it is easily solved by separation of variables. All that is needed is an initial condition. This is provided by the fact that at time t = 0 when the model begins, the initial number of infectives is $I(0) = I_o$. Separating and integrating leads to

$$\int_{I_o}^{I(t)} d\tilde{I}/\tilde{I} = B \int_0^t d\tilde{t}$$

thus

$$I(t) = I_o \exp\{Bt\}$$

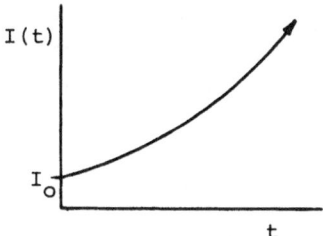

The basic defect of the model is easily seen from the graph above. As time passes, the number of infectives is seen to grow without bound. This property is easily traced to the initial premise on which the model is based. Specifically, that the population at risk of catching the disease is effectively infinite in size. A more realistic model will take into account that there are only a finite number of susceptible individuals.

II. The Classical Simple Epidemic Model

To overcome the problem encountered in the previous model, it is next assumed that at all times the population under consideration numbers N individuals. Everyone in the population is either susceptible to the disease or else infected with the disease.

In addition to the variables defined for the previous model, let:

$S(t)$ = number of susceptible individuals at time t

β = average number of contacts between susceptible and infected individuals which lead to a new infective per unit of time per infective per susceptible in the population.

n.b. By comparing the definitions of B and β it should be clear that $B = \beta S(t)$. Although B was treated as a constant in the first model, it is now seen to vary with the number of susceptibles.

Since the total population size never entered into the derivation of the equation for the number of infectives in the first model, the same argument with B replaced by $\beta S(t)$ leads to

$$\frac{dI(t)}{dt} = \beta S(t) I(t)$$

In addition, since the total population size is always N, and since all individuals are either susceptible or infected,

$$S(t) + I(t) = N$$

n.b. It is simple to derive the governing differential equation for the number of susceptibles. From an argument similar to the one which lead to the differential equation for $I(t)$ in the first model, or more directly by differentiating the definition of the constant total population size with respect to time and using the equation for $I(t)$, it follows that

$$\frac{dS(t)}{dt} = -\beta S(t) I(t)$$

However, since $S(t)$ can be eliminated using $S(t) = N - I(t)$ in the differential equation for $I(t)$, one need only solve

$$\frac{dI(t)}{dt} = \beta I(t) [N - I(t)]$$

Although this differential equation is nonlinear, it submits to the same method of solution as the linear differential equation in the previous section. As before, the initial number of infectives is $I(0) = I_o$, where $0 < I_o \leq N$, and typically, $I_o \ll N$. Separating variables leads to

$$\int_{I_o}^{I(t)} \frac{d\tilde{I}}{\tilde{I}(N - \tilde{I})} = \beta \int_0^t d\tilde{t}$$

Expanding the denominator of the integrand on the left-hand side using partial fractions, integrating and rearranging provides

$$I(t) = \frac{I_o \exp\{N\beta t\}}{1 - \frac{I_o}{N}(1 - \exp\{N\beta t\})}$$

It is informative to look at the limiting behavior of this solution:

1. In the limit as $N \to \infty$ the denominator becomes unity and (with the proviso that $\beta N \to B$) the solution is identical with the solution to the first model.

2. In the limit as $t \to \infty$, since $N > 0$ and $\beta > 0$, the exponentials dominate both the numerator and the denominator, so $I(t) \to N$.

Taken together, these two asymptotic observations suggest that in a large population with a small initial number of infectives, at first the epidemic (as measured by the total number of infectives) grows exponentially. Then, as fewer susceptibles are available, the rate of growth decreases, but the epidemic does not end until everyone in the population has contracted the disease.

A typical solution as a function of time is shown in the figure on the next page:

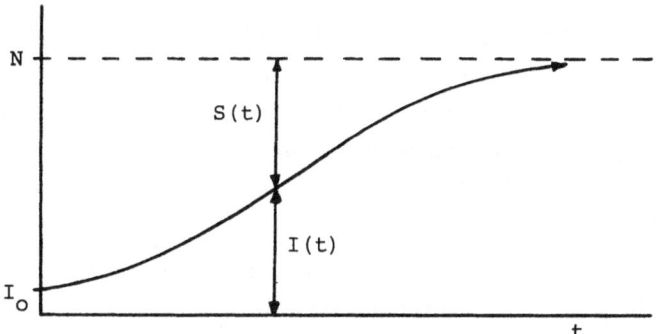

Although the analytic form of I(t) is now known, and a similar
expression for S(t) follows immediately from the fact that $S(t) = N - I(t)$,
in practice these are not the observed quantities in a epidemic.   The
more usual quantity to report is the 'epidemic curve' which records the
rate at which the disease spreads in the population.   For the present
model the epidemic curve, W(t), is the rate of change in the number of
infectives, thus

$$W(t) = \frac{dI(t)}{dt} = \beta S(t) I(t)$$

$$= \frac{\beta (N - I_o) I_o \exp\{N\beta t\}}{[1 - \frac{I_o}{N}(1 - \exp\{N\beta t\})]^2}$$

Typically, this function looks like:

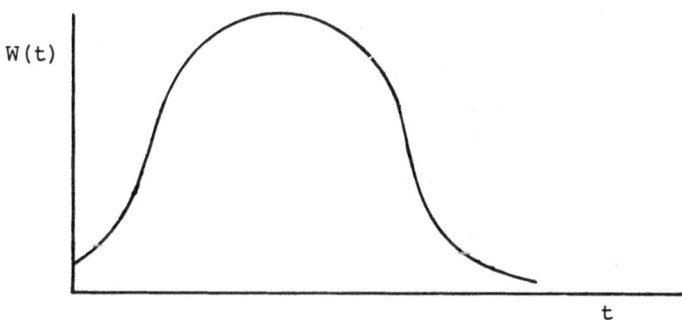

n.b.   It is not difficult to show that W(t) is symmetrical about its
       maximum.

The second model is considerably better than the first, but still has
one rather unrealistic aspect.   Notice that whenever an epidemic gets
started, everyone in the population ultimately contracts the disease.
The reason for this can be traced to the fact that infectives remain
infected forever.   A more realistic model must take into account that
for most diseases infectives either recover or else they die.

III. The Classical General Epidemic Model (Kermack-McKendrick)

In order to overcome the problem encountered in the previous model, it is assumed that infectives are removed from circulation at a rate which is proportional to the current number of infectives. Since for many diseases a natural immunity occurs, it is further assumed that former infectives enter a new class which is not susceptible to the disease.

n.b. By introducing a class of removed individuals, we have managed to avoid a precise statement of the severity of the disease being modeled. The removals may be recovered and immune, or they may be quarantined and thus out of circulation or they may be dead. All that is necessary is that the disease not be available to any individual more than once.

In addition to the variables defined in the previous models, let:

$R(t)$ = number of removed individuals at time t

γ = average rate of removal of infectives from circulation per unit time per infective in the population.

Since the new class of individuals, the removals, in no way interacts with the susceptibles, the governing equation for the susceptibles is unchanged from the second model. Thus the differential equation is

$$\frac{dS(t)}{dt} = -\beta\, S(t)\, I(t)$$

The differential equation developed previously for the number of infectives must be modified to take into account the removals. Using an argument similar to the one for the first model considered, it is not hard to deduce the equation

$$\frac{dI(t)}{dt} = \beta\, S(t)\, I(t) - \gamma\, I(t)$$

The individuals who are removed from the ranks of the infectives then contribute to the number of removed individuals according to the relation

$$\frac{dR(t)}{dt} = \gamma\, I(t)$$

Since all individuals in the population are either susceptible, infected or removed, it follows that since the population is constant in size,

$$S(t) + I(t) + R(t) = N$$

n.b.   By differentiating this last expression with respect to time, it
       follows that the sum of the three governing equations must sum
       to zero (as they in fact do.)   In addition, the last expression
       guarantees that once the size of any two of the classes is known,
       the size of the third follows by simple arithmetic.

To complete the specification of the model it is necessary to know the
initial state of the population.   Assume that at time $t = 0$ there are
no removed individuals, a very small number, I_o, of infectives, and
the remainder of the population, S_o, is susceptible.   Thus,

$$S(0) = S_o = N - I_o; \quad I(0) = I_o << N; \quad R(0) = 0$$

Before attempting to find a solution to the set of governing equations,
it is informative to look carefully at the equations.   Specifically,
look at the equation for the number of infectives in the form

$$\frac{dI(t)}{dt} = \beta [S(t) - \rho] I(t) : \quad \rho \equiv \gamma/\beta$$

Clearly, since $I(t) \geq 0$, the sign of the term in square brackets is the
same as the sign of $dI(t)/dt$, hence

$$\frac{dI(t)}{dt} > 0 \quad \text{if and only if} \quad S(t) > \rho$$

Further, since $S(t)$ is a monotonically decreasing function of time
(since susceptibles become infected and no new susceptibles are made)
if $S(0) < \rho$ then $S(t) < \rho$ for all $t > 0$ and $dI(t)/dt < 0$ for all
future time.   In other words, if the initial number of susceptibles is
smaller than some critical number, ρ, there will not be an epidemic
(where here the word epidemic is used in the technical sense of a
large, one-time outbreak of the disease.)

We proceed now to analyze the model in detail.   To do so, begin by
eliminating the explicit dependence on $I(t)$ between the first and the
third of the governing differential equation to get

$$\frac{dS(t)}{dt} = - \frac{S(t)}{\rho} \frac{dR(t)}{dt}$$

Separating variables, multiplying through by dt and integrating leads
to

$$S(t) = S_o \exp\{-R(t)/\rho\}$$

Next, make use of the relation $S(t) + I(t) + R(t) = N$ in the equation
for $R(t)$:

$$\frac{dR(t)}{dt} = \gamma I(t) = \gamma [N - R(t) - S(t)]$$

and then use the expression just derived to eliminate S(t); thus

$$\frac{dR(t)}{dt} = \gamma [N - R(t) - S_o \exp\{-R(t)/\rho\}]$$

Note that R(t) is the only one of the dependent variables which appears in this equation. Although it is possible to solve this differential equation exactly, the methods are rather complicated. We therefore seek and approximate solution.

Since this difficulty in solving the equation results from the presence of the exponential term, we proceed to replace the exponentials by a polynomial. To do so we expand the exponential in a Taylor Series about the only point at which we know the value of R(t). Specifically, we expand about R(0) = 0; this leads to:

$$\exp\{-R(t)/\rho\} = 1 - \left(\frac{R(t)}{\rho}\right) + \frac{1}{2} \left(\frac{R(t)}{\rho}\right)^2 - \frac{1}{6} \left(\frac{R(t)}{\rho}\right)^3 + \cdots$$

Clearly, if one attempts to retain the entire infinite series, nothing has been gained. By truncating the series after the first few terms, a separable differential equation which is fairly easily solved will result. The question remains, how many terms should be retained ? It is not difficult to show that if only terms up to the linear one are kept, only an absurd answer is possible. On the other hand, if terms up to the cubic one are kept, the resulting integration is very hard. We therefore choose to keep terms up to the quadratic one, thereby balancing realism against solvability. Following a bit of rearranging, the resulting equation is:

$$\frac{dR(t)}{dt} = \gamma [I_o + (\frac{S_o}{\rho} - 1) R(t) - \frac{S_o}{2\rho^2} R(t)^2]$$

Separating variables and integrating leads to the expression:

$$R(t) = \frac{\rho^2}{S_o} \left[\frac{S_o}{\rho} - 1 + \alpha \tanh(\frac{\alpha\gamma t}{2} - \phi) \right]$$

where

$$\alpha = \sqrt{\left(\frac{S_o}{\rho} - 1\right)^2 + 2S_o I_o/\rho^2}$$

$$\phi = \tanh^{-1}[(\frac{S_o}{\rho} - 1)/\alpha]$$

n.b. Developing this solution is straightforward, but does involve a considerable amount of rather messy algebra.

As with the second model, we are really more interested in knowing the shape of the predicted epidemic curve, W(t), than the cumulative number of removals, R(t). Since cases of the disease are counted as victims seek medical attention, and this is also the time at which individuals are removed from active circulation, it is customary to assume that

$$W(t) = \frac{dR(t)}{dt} = \frac{\gamma \alpha^2 \rho^2}{2S_o} \operatorname{sech}^2 (\frac{\alpha \gamma t}{2} - \phi)$$

Note that this expression describes a function which rises to a single
maximum at time $t = 2\phi/\alpha\gamma$ and then dies away symmetrically. This is
very similar to the result for the epidemic curve in the second model;
however, in this model not all susceptibles need to be infected as we
will now see.

We wish to look at the asymptotic behavior of the epidemic as $t \to \infty$.
Since there are only a finite number of individuals in the population
and since none can contract the disease more than once, the epidemic
must eventually die out. Further, once the epidemic has ended, all
individuals will be either still susceptible or else removed. None are
still infected. We therefore look at the quantity

$$\lim_{t \to \infty} R(t) \equiv R_\infty = \frac{\rho^2}{S_o} \left[\frac{S_o}{\rho} - 1 + \alpha \right]$$

If it is further assumed that the epidemic is started by a very small
group of infectives, so that

$$2S_o I_o/\rho^2 \ll \frac{S_o}{\rho} - 1 \quad : \quad S_o > \rho$$

it then follows from the definition of α that

$$\alpha \approx \frac{S_o}{\rho} - 1$$

and
$$R_\infty \approx 2\rho (1 - \frac{\rho}{S_o})$$

The condition for an epidemic outbreak of the disease is $S_o > \rho$. Assume
that $S_o = \rho + \epsilon$, where $0 < \epsilon \ll \rho$. Substitute this into the equation
for R_∞ to get

$$R_\infty = 2\rho (\frac{\epsilon}{\rho + \epsilon}) \approx 2\epsilon$$

This means that for a population which initially has $S_o = \rho + \epsilon$
susceptibles, after the epidemic has subsided, there will be about
$S_\infty = \rho - \epsilon$ susceptibles remaining. In other words, the final number
of susceptibles is as far below the threshold for an epidemic as the
initial number was above the threshold. This result is called the
Kermack-McKendrick Threshold Theorem.

n.b. Instead of starting by letting $t \to \infty$ in $R(t)$, we could have noted
     that in the limit, $dR(t)/dt = 0$. Thus, by setting the right-hand
     side of the differential equation for $R(t)$ equal to zero, we could

have deduced the Kermack-McKendrick Threshold Theorem without ever finding R(t) explicitly.

Problems

1. Assume that in the first model discussed, B = B(t), so that

$$\frac{dI(t)}{dt} = B(t)I(t) \quad ; \quad I(0) = I_o$$

Find the solution to this differential equation.

2. Work through the details of finding the solution to the second model

$$\frac{dI(t)}{dt} = \beta I(t)[N - I(t)] \quad : \quad I(0) = I_o$$

Note: No tables allowed - use partial fractions instead.

3. For the second model, find the time at which the epidemic curve, W(t), achieves its maximum, and show that W(t) is symmetric about that time:

$$W(t) = \frac{\beta(N - I_o)I_o \exp\{N\beta t\}}{[1 - \frac{I_o}{N}(1 - \exp\{N\beta t\})]^2}$$

4. Show that if only the linear terms are kept in the approximate form of the differential equation for R(t) in the third model, the solution which results is nonsense. The equation to be solved takes the form:

$$\frac{dR(t)}{dt} = \gamma[I_o + (\frac{S_o}{\rho} - 1)R(t)] \quad : \quad R(0) = 0$$

Hint: One way to proceed is to shift the origin of the dependent variable in order to transform the equation to a familiar form.

5. Work through the details of finding the solution to the third model in its approximate form

$$\frac{dR(t)}{dt} = \gamma[I_o + (\frac{S_o}{\rho} - 1) R(t) - \frac{S_o}{2\rho^2} R(t)^2] \quad : \quad R(0) = 0$$

Note: No tables allowed - complete the square and make a hyperbolic trigonometric substitutuion. Assume that $S_o > \rho$.

6. Assuming that you know R(t) (at least in its approximate form) for the third model, determine I(t) and S(t) to the same degree of approximation. Plot typical shapes for the three functions against time.

Hint: This is an easy problem - stop and think before you become involved in lots of unnecessary algebra.

References

The material in this section can be found in virtually any text on mathematical epidemiology, as well as in a number of books on mathematical modeling. Two useful books are:

Bailey, N.T.J., The Mathematical Theory of Infectious Diseases, Hafner Press, New York, 1975.

> This is probably the most comprehensive book on the subject of mathematical epidemiology. The second and third models of the present chapter are discussed in detail in sections 5.1 - 5.2 and 6.1 - 6.2, respectively.

Maki, D.P. and M. Thompson, Mathematical Models and Applications, Prentice-Hall, Englewood Cliffs, N.J., 1973.

> In sections 9.0 - 9.1, the second and third models of the present chapter are discussed. The level of treatment is about the same as here.

Chapter 2. Rumors and Mousetraps

In this section two unrelated mathematical models are discussed. While neither model is specifically concerned with an epidemic of a contagious disease, both are abstractions of classical models of epidemics. The first model is concerned with the spread of a rumor through a group of loosely connected communities, the second with a stylized simulation of a chain reaction. In order to help emphasize the similarity to epidemic models, the customary variable names in epidemiology will be employed throughout.

The Discrete Time Spread of a Rumor

We consider a group of N + 1 isolated small villages which can only communicate with one another by means of an archaic telephone system. The phone system permits one pair of villages to be in contact at any time, one village making the call, the other village receiving the call. The rumor is spread by means of these telephone calls, and an entire village is considered to know the rumor once the village receives it.

The N + 1 villages fall into three types:

   S (Susceptible): Villages which have not yet heard the rumor, but which would be interested in spreading it to other villages once it is known.

   I (Infective): Villages which have heard the rumor and are active in spreading it to other villages.

   R (Removed): Villages which have previously heard the rumor, but which are no longer interested in spreading it to other villages.

The dynamics for the spread of the rumor are assumed to be as follows:

1. When the telephone lines are free, a randomly selected village (of any type) places a call. The call is then connected at random to any of the other N villages, again without regard for type (S, I or R).

2. If a village of type I calls a village of type S, the rumor (infection) is spread. Consequently, both villages become of type I.

3. If a village of type I calls a village of either type I or type R, the village making the call loses interest in the rumor and becomes of type R. The village receiving the call does not change type.

4. Calls emanating from villages of either type S or type R have no effect, and hence are meaningless as far as the rumor spread is concerned.

n.b. It therefore follows that we really only need concern ourselves with calls of the sort described in items 2 and 3; all calls which alter the state of the system emanate from villages of type I.

We assume that as the model starts, there is one village of type I which knows the rumor and the other N villages are of type S.

In constructing the mathematical model the first problem which must be addressed is the treatment of time. One obvious but not entirely satisfactory method is to assume that time is discrete and integer valued such that the time index increases by one each time a village of type I completes a call. Hence, let time be denoted by $t = 0, 1, 2, \ldots$

n.b. While this specification is convenient internally (within the model) it has no obvious relation to time in the real world. To create a correspondence, one must consider the frequency of calls made by villages of type I as a function of the state of the model.

Specifying the dependent variable presents an even greater problem, as there is uncertainty in just how the rumor spreads. Temporarily, ignore this difficulty and define the 'condition vector'

$$\underset{\rightarrow}{P}(t) = [s(t), i(t), r(t)]$$

where $s(t)$, $i(t)$ and $r(t)$ are the number of villages of types S, I and R, respectively, at time t. Clearly, from the initial state defined above,

$$\underset{\rightarrow}{P}(0) = [N, 1, 0]$$

The first call which changes the state of the system (whenever it occurs in real time) causes the time index to increase to t = 1, and consists of having the one village of type I (which knows the rumor) call one of the N villages of type S. Thus,

$$\underset{\rightarrow}{P}(1) = [N-1,2,0]$$

At this point the difficulty anticipated above becomes apparent. There are now two different types of calls which alter the state of the model which are possible: one of the two type I villages can call one of the N-1 type S villages, or one of the two type I villages can call the other type I village. The precise state of the system is uncertain for t ≥ 2.

To avoid the difficulty of keeping track of the probability of all of the different possible outcomes, we choose to work with an expectation-like variable. In fact, for t = 2 it is precisely the expectation:

$$\underset{\rightarrow 2}{P} \equiv E[\underset{\rightarrow}{P}(t=2)] \equiv [s_2, i_2, r_2]$$

and for t = k = 3, 4, ...

$$\underset{\rightarrow k}{P} \equiv E[\underset{\rightarrow}{P}(t=k) | \underset{\rightarrow}{P}(t=k-1) = \underset{\rightarrow k-1}{P}] \equiv [s_k, i_k, r_k]$$

n.b. The idea is that for k = 3, 4, ... we calculate the vector $\underset{\rightarrow k}{P}$ recursively, assuming that we know the true vector $\underset{\rightarrow}{P}(t=k-1)$. In reality, all we know it its expectation-like value $\underset{\rightarrow k-1}{P}$. Note also that s_k, i_k and r_k are generally not integers.

We next develop the recurrence relations which constitute the model. To do so, assume that at t = k-1 we know that $\underset{\rightarrow k-1}{P} = [s_{k-1}, i_{k-1}, r_{k-1}]$. The actual state $\underset{\rightarrow}{P}(t=k)$ is then either

$$[s_{k-1} - 1, i_{k-1} + 1, r_{k-1}] \text{ or } [s_{k-1}, i_{k-1} - 1, r_{k-1} + 1]$$

where the first form results if a village of type I calls a village of type S, which occurs with probability s_{k-1}/N, and the second form results if a village of type I calls either a village of type I or type R, which occurs with probability $(N - s_{k-1})/N$. Consequently, the first two elements of the vector $\underset{\rightarrow k}{P}$ are:

$$s_k = \frac{s_{k-1}}{N} (s_{k-1} - 1) + \frac{N - s_{k-1}}{N} (s_{k-1}) = \frac{N - 1}{N} s_{k-1}$$

$$i_k = \frac{s_{k-1}}{N} (i_{k-1} + 1) + \frac{N - s_{k-1}}{N} (i_{k-1} - 1)$$

$$= i_{k-1} + \frac{2}{N} s_{k-1} - 1$$

n.b.   Both these equations are clearly valid for k = 0, 1, 2, ...
        Also, since $s_k + i_k + r_k = N + 1$, it is not necessary to write
        down the recurrence relation for r_k explicitly.

We proceed next to find solutions to the two recurrence relations which
are seen to be a pair of coupled linear difference equations. Look at
the equation for s_k first; it is readily solved by induction:

$$s_1 = \frac{N - 1}{N} \, s_0$$

$$s_2 = \frac{N - 1}{N} \, s_1 = \left(\frac{N - 1}{N}\right)^2 \, s_0$$

$$\vdots$$

$$s_k = \frac{N - 1}{N} \, s_{k-1} = \cdots = \left(\frac{N - 1}{N}\right)^k \, s_0 = N\left(\frac{N - 1}{N}\right)^k$$

Once s_k is known, i_k is found easily as follows:

$$i_1 - i_0 = 2\left(\frac{N - 1}{N}\right)^0 - 1$$

$$i_2 - i_1 = 2\left(\frac{N - 1}{N}\right)^1 - 1$$

$$\vdots$$

$$i_k - i_{k-1} = 2\left(\frac{N - 1}{N}\right)^{k-1} - 1$$

Adding these k equations together on both sides of the equal sign yields:

$$i_k - i_0 = 2\sum_{j=0}^{k-1}\left(\frac{N - 1}{N}\right)^j - k$$

n.b.   Recall that $i_0 = 1$, and

$$\sum_{j=0}^{k-1} x^j = \frac{1 - x^k}{1 - x}$$

Hence

$$i_k = 2N\left[1 - \left(1 - \frac{1}{N}\right)^k\right] + 1 - k \quad : \quad k = 0, 1, 2, \ldots$$

This completes the solution to the basic model. The solution consists
of explicit formulas for s_k and i_k and the definition $r_k = N - 1 - s_k - i_k$.
For any choice of N it is simple to find the evolution of the rumor in
time. However, this does not give any very general result about the
most interesting question:

How Far does the Rumor Get ?

Clearly, the rumor is over once there are no more villages of type I.

We will seek as an answer to our question the number of villages of type S which remain when no type I villages are left. Thus we wish to know the value of k for which $i_k = 0$.

n.b. Since the i_k are not in general integer valued, we would expect to find $i_m > 0$ and $i_{m+1} < 0$. To get around this difficulty, we will replace k by λN in the equation for i_k, and treat λ as a continuous variable. Hence we will look for the value of λ that causes $i_{\lambda N} = 0$.

Setting the expression for i_k from above equal to zero yields:

$$0 = 2N \left[1 - \left(1 - \frac{1}{N} \right)^{\lambda N} \right] + 1 - \lambda N$$

thus

$$\lambda = 2 - 2 \left[\left(1 - \frac{1}{N} \right)^N \right]^\lambda + \frac{1}{N}$$

If N is large, this equation can be solved rather easily. In the limit as $N \to \infty$:

$$\frac{1}{N} \to 0 \quad \text{and} \quad \left(1 - \frac{1}{N} \right)^N \to \exp\{-1\}$$

Thus $\lambda \to \lambda *$, a constant satisfying the expression

$$\lambda * = 2 - 2\exp\{-\lambda *\}$$

$$\equiv g(\lambda *)$$

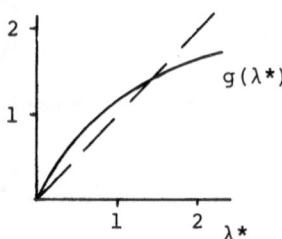

This transcendential equation can be seen from the figure to the right to have just one root. It is easily found by trial and error to be, $\lambda * \approx 1.594$

It therefore follows that the rumor dies out after about $t = \lambda * N = 1.594N$ telephone calls by type I villages when N is large, and further, since

$$s_{\lambda N} = N \left(\frac{N - 1}{N} \right)^{\lambda N}$$

when N is large,

$$s_{\lambda * N} \approx N \exp\{-\lambda *\} = 0.238N$$

Hence, when the rumor dies out, about 23.8% of the villages will not have heard it.

In the process of finding the duration of the rumor, an number of rather cavalier assumptions were made without very much justification. It therefore seems wise to confirm our approximate solution. Since the analytic form of the solution is known, this is simple to do by trial and error. In the table below we list the value of m, where $i_m > 0$ and $i_{m+1} < 0$, along with the implied value of $\lambda * \approx m/N$, for several values of N.

N	m	m/N
10	17	1.700
100	161	1.610
1000	1595	1.595

Since our approximate method led to the conclusion that for large N, $\lambda*$ → 1.594, we conclude that our method appears to be correct.

n.b.   In the process of formulating the model we made another important
approximation; specifically, we assumed that we could replace the
condition vector by an expectation-like quantity. Although no
good justification or method of validation appears to be available,
one potential risk inherent to this simplification is explained in
an appendix at the end of this chapter.

The Mousetrap Chain Reaction

Imagine that the floor of a room is covered with N mousetraps, and that
k ping-pong balls are placed upon the bail of each trap. A ball is then
thrown into the room to start the process. Under certain conditions, a
'chain reaction' will ensue. We will now build a mathematical model to
describe the process.

We begin by making a number of assumptions:

1.   The flight time for each ball is the same, and equal to
one unit of time.

2.   If a ball hits an unsprung trap, the trap is set-off, and
the ball which sprung the trap comes to rest.

3.   If a ball hits a trap which has already been sprung, the
ball comes immediately to rest.

Choose as the independent variable time t, measured in units of flight
time, so t = 0, 1, 2, ... Also, let:

S(t) = number of unsprung traps remaining after the event at
time t = 0, 1, 2, ... ; thus, S(0) = N.

J(t) = number of balls in the air in the time interval which
begins at time t = 0, 1, 2, ... ; thus, J(0) = 1.

n.b.   To continue the analogy with the epidemic models, we should also
define:

I(t) = J(t)/k for t = 1, 2, 3, ... , where k is the number of
balls per trap and I(0) is undefined since the first
ball which starts the reaction is introduced from

outside of the system.

$$R(t) = N - S(t) - I(t)$$

Since the ball which starts the reaction is certain to hit an unsprung trap, it follows immediately that

$$J(1) = k$$

and

$$S(1) = N - J(1)/k = N - 1$$

n.b.   Hence, $I(1) = 1$ and $R(1) = 0$.

In attempting to continue to the second time epoch we encounter the same difficulty as in the model for the spread of a rumor. Specifically, $S(t)$ and $J(t)$ are really integer-valued random variables which have probability densities which are complicated functions of time.

In an effort to keep the model simple, we choose to work with a set of expectation-like variables:

$$J_n = E[J(t=n)|J(t=n-1)=J_{n-1}]$$

and

$$S_n = N - \frac{1}{k} \sum_{i=1}^{n} J_i$$

n.b.   Once again, to complete the analogy with epidemic models, it follows that $I_n = J_n/k$ and since $S_n + I_n + R_n = N$,

$$R_n = \frac{1}{k} \sum_{i=1}^{n-1} J_i$$

The next step is to relate J_n to J_{n-1} and S_{n-1}. To do so, assume that the probability of hitting an unsprung trap equals the fraction of unsprung traps remaining, which is just S_{n-1}/N, so

$$J_n = k J_{n-1} S_{n-1}/N = k J_{n-1}\left[1 - \frac{1}{kN} \sum_{i=1}^{n-1} J_i\right]$$

This equation is a nonlinear difference equation; unfortunately, it can not be solved analytically.

n.b.   Since we know that $J_1 = k$, for any choices of k and N it is a simple operation to evaluate recursively $J_2, J_3, \ldots$.

In order to proceed, it is convenient to convert the governing equation to a form in which the summation does not appear explicitly. To do so, recall that

$$R_n = \frac{1}{k} \sum_{i=1}^{n-1} J_i$$

and thus

$$R_{n+1} - R_n = \frac{1}{k} J_n$$

Using these relations in the nonlinear difference equation leads to the equivalent form:

$$R_{n+1} - R_n = k(R_n - R_{n-1})(1 - R_n/N)$$

which following division of both sides by N can be rearranged into the form:

$$Z_{n+1} - 2Z_n + Z_{n-1} = (Z_n - Z_{n-1})[(k-1) - kZ_n]$$

where

$$Z_n = R_n/N = \text{average fraction of traps sprung prior}$$
$$\text{to time } t = n.$$

The next transformation is rather unusual. Since it is easier to deal with nonlinear differential equations than with nonlinear difference equations, we introduce a continuous variable $Z(x)$, defined such that $Z(x=n) = Z_n$. In addition, we define the function at $x = n+1$ and $x = n-1$ by means of the Taylor Series expansion about the point $x = n$:

$$Z_{n\pm1} = Z(x=n\pm1) = Z(x=n) \pm \left.\frac{dZ}{dx}\right|_{x=n} + \left.\frac{d^2Z}{dx^2}\right|_{x=n} \pm \cdots$$

Substituting into the difference equation and discarding terms which are third derivatives or higher leads to the differential equation

$$\frac{d^2Z}{dx^2} = \left[\frac{dZ}{dx} - \frac{1}{2}\frac{d^2Z}{dx^2}\right][(k-1) - kZ]$$

n.b. We have dropped the 'evaluated at x=n' as we want the differential
      equation to represent the behavior for all continuous values of x.

Introducing the shorthand notation $(\cdot)' \equiv d(\cdot)/dx$, and rearranging the differential equation leads to:

$$Z'' = 2Z' - \frac{4Z'}{(k+1) - kZ}$$

This equation can be integrated directly to yield:

$$Z' = 2Z + \frac{4}{k} \ln\left[1 - \frac{k}{k+1}Z\right] + C$$

where C is a constant of integration. To evaluate this constant notice that at $x = 1$, $Z(1) = R(1)/N = 0$ and $Z'(1) \simeq [R(2)-R(1)]/N = 1/N$; thus $C \simeq 1/N$.

Although it is not simple to integrate the differential equation again, it is possible at this point to extract an interesting result. Observe that at the end of the experiment, $Z' = 0$, hence

$$2Z_e + \frac{4}{k} \ln\left[1 - \frac{k}{k+1} Z_e\right] + \frac{1}{N} = 0$$

where Z_e is the value of $Z(x)$ at the end of the experiment. Since $N \gg 1$, $1/N \simeq 0$; thus

$$Z_e \simeq -\frac{2}{k} \ln\left[1 - \frac{k}{k+1} Z_e\right]$$

This is a transcendential equation which is easily solved by trial and error. At integer values of k one finds:

k	Z_e
1	4.5×10^{-6}
2	0.87
3	1.06

n.b. Since Z_e can in theory never exceed unity, the final entry in the table serves to remind us that our solution is approximate.

Since k represents the number of balls per trap, one would expect k to be an integer. However, if k is thought of as a continuous variable, then the system exhibits a threshold-like behavior which depends upon whether k < 1 or k > 1; this is apparent from the figure below.

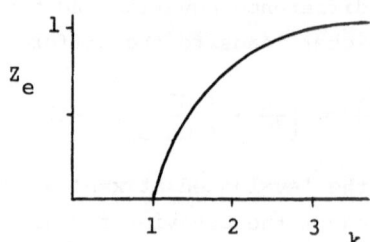

Notice that the value of Z_e, which represents the fraction of traps which are sprung after the experiment ends, rises very sharply as k increases from 1 to 2.

Maximum Number of Traps Sprung in any Time Epoch

We begin by introducing the continuous variable I(x) defined such that $I(x=n) = I_n$. It then follows that $Z'(x) \simeq I(x)/N$. Next, recall that if k > 1, a 'chain reaction' occurs. At the time x* when the maximum number of traps go off, $I(x*) = I_{max}$, and thus $I'(x*) = 0$. It is not difficult to show that at this time, $Z(x*) = (k-1)/k$.

It then follows from the once integrated form of the differential equation evaluated at x = x*:

$$Z'(x*) = \frac{I_{max}}{N} \simeq 2Z(x*) + \frac{4}{k} \ln\left[1 - \frac{k}{k+1} Z(x*)\right]$$

that the maximum number of traps sprung in any one time epoch is

$$I_{max} \cong \frac{N}{k}\left[2(k-1) + 4\ln\left(\frac{2}{k+1}\right)\right]$$

As a function of continuous k, this look like

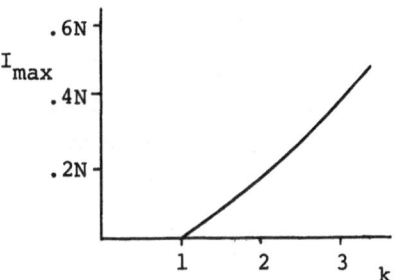

Thus, as the number of balls per trap increases, the strength of the 'chain reaction' as measured by the maximum fraction of traps sprung at the height of the reaction increases.

Time History of the 'Chain Reaction'

The trajectory of the reaction in time is found by integrating the once integrated differential equation a second time. Upon separating the variables, it is found that the form is

$$\int_0^z \frac{d\tilde{z}}{\frac{1}{N} + 2\tilde{z} + \frac{4}{k}\ln\left[1 - \frac{k}{k+1}\tilde{z}\right]} = \int_1^x d\tilde{x} = x - 1$$

Since this is not easily integrated, expand the logarithm in a series near to $\tilde{z} = 0$:

$$\ln\left[1 - \frac{k}{k+1}\tilde{z}\right] = -\frac{k}{k+1}\tilde{z} - \frac{1}{2}\left(\frac{k}{k+1}\tilde{z}\right)^2 + \cdots$$

However, if we simply truncate this series after the quadratic term, the approximation violates the relation employed to evaluate z_e:

$$z_e \cong -\frac{2}{k}\ln\left[1 - \frac{k}{k+1}z_e\right]$$

We therefore adjust the constant on the quadratic term in the series expansion so that this relation holds also, and employ:

$$\ln\left[1 - \frac{k}{k+1}\tilde{z}\right] \cong -\frac{k}{k+1}\tilde{z} - \frac{k(k-1)}{2(k+1)}\frac{\tilde{z}^2}{z_e}$$

hence the integral becomes:

$$\frac{k+1}{2(k-1)}\int_0^y \frac{d\tilde{y}}{c + \tilde{y} + \tilde{y}^2} = x - 1$$

where $y = Z/Z_e$ and $C = (k+1)/[2(k-1)NZ_e]$.

n.b. This integral is still not simple, and in fact leads to results in terms of the hyperbolic tangent. A further approximation is however possible.

Look at the denominator of the integrand:

$$C + \tilde{y} + \tilde{y}^2 = (\tilde{y}_1 - \tilde{y})(\tilde{y} - \tilde{y}_2) \approx (1 + C - \tilde{y})(\tilde{y} + C)$$

since $C \ll 1$. Employing partial fractions, and the approximation that $\tilde{y}_1 + \tilde{y}_2 \approx \tilde{y}_1 - \tilde{y}_2 \approx 1$ in the integration leads to the parametric form for the trajectory:

$$\left(\frac{1 + C}{C}\right)\left(\frac{y + C}{1 + C - y}\right) = \exp\{2(k-1)(x-1)/(k+1)\}$$

n.b. y represents the fraction of the traps which will ever be sprung which are sprung at time x. If one plots y against x, it turns out that as x increases, y first increases slowly, then more quickly, and then slowly again. A curve of this form, which was encountered in the second epidemic model, is sometimes called a 'logistic' curve.

Time to the End of the Experiment

At the end of the experiment, $y = 1$ and $x = x_e$. To evaluate x_e we set $y = 1$ in the expression above to get:

$$\left(\frac{1 + C}{C}\right)^2 \approx \left(\frac{1}{C}\right)^2 = \exp\{2(k-1)(x_e-1)/(k+1)\}$$

Hence,

$$x_e \approx 1 + \frac{k+1}{k-1} \ln\left[\frac{2(k-1)NZ_e}{(k+1)}\right]$$

Thus, for example, if $k = 2$, and hence $Z_e \approx 0.87$, we find the following results for the duration of an experiment:

N	x_e
100	13.2
1000	20.1
10000	27.0

n.b. The duration of the reaction increases rather slowly with increasing numbers of traps.

Appendix

In both of the models considered in this chapter, the computation of the behavior of a random variable was replaced by the calculation of sequentially conditioned expected values of the variable. While this

device greatly simplified the mathematics, it is important to realize
the potential risk inherent to such a procedure.

Consider the following (contrived) example for which the expected value
is a terribly misleading estimate of the actual behavior.

Let X be a random variable which takes on just two values as follows:

$$\text{Prob}\{X = N^2\} = 1/N$$
$$\text{Prob}\{X = 0\} = (N-1)/N$$

Thus, $E(X) = N^2 \cdot (1/N) + 0 \cdot (N-1)/N = N$

Consequently, as $N \to \infty$, the expected value of X grows without bound,
yet the probability that $X = 0$ approaches unity.

n.b.   It should be clear that what is happening is that the expected
       value is averaging an extremely likely value of zero with an
       extremely unlikely huge number, and coming up with something in
       between which does not represent either outcome.

Some insight into the source of the problem is provided by finding the
variance.

$$V(X) = E(X^2) - E(X)^2$$

Since $E(X^2) = N^4 \cdot (1/N) + \cdot 0^2 \cdot (N-1)/N = N^3$

$$V(X) = N^3 - N^2 = N^2(N-1)$$

and thus the standard deviation is

$$\sqrt{V(X)} = N\sqrt{N-1}$$

The thing to notice is that the standard deviation grows faster than
the mean as N gets large. Ordinarily, when this happens, the expected
value is not a good estimate of the behavior. However, without some
estimate of the variance it is impossible to predict whether the results
being found are meaningless. But to calculate the variance, it is
necessary to calculate the probabilities for the random variable. Thus
it is impossible to assess the accuracy of the results for the rumor
model or the mousetrap model.

Problems

1. Suggest a mechanism for relating model time to clock time in the
    rumor model. Use this mechanism to construct a mathematical model
    for estimating the clock time duration of a rumor and carry out the
    solution as far as you are able.

2. With $\underset{\to k}{P} = (s_k, i_k, r_k)$ as defined in the rumor model, derive an
    expression for r_k, and show that $s_k + i_k + r_k = N + 1$.

3. Find an approximate expression for the size of the error which is introduced when the expression:

$$\lambda = 2 - 2 \left[\left(1 - \frac{1}{N} \right)^N \right]^\lambda + \frac{1}{N}$$

is replaced by $\lambda^* \simeq 2 - 2 \exp \{-\lambda^*\}$. Your answer should be a series (polynomial) in powers of N. Find the coefficient of the leading term.

4. Devise a first order iterative scheme to estimate the root of

$$\lambda^* = 2 - 2 \exp \{-\lambda^*\}$$

Hint: If this question sounds unfamiliar, try looking up the Newton-Raphson method in a book on numerical methods.

5. Starting with the differential equation for the mousetrap problem:

$$Z'' = 2Z' - \frac{4Z'}{(k+1) - kZ}$$

estimate the short-time behavior of the solution (when $Z \simeq 0$).

6. If $I(x^*) = I_{max}$, show that $Z(x^*) = (k-1)/k$.

References

The two models discussed in this chapter find their origins in the educational and not the technical literature. As such, clear and well written expositions are to be found in the original sources which are listed below:

Carrier, G.F., Topics in Applied Mathematics, Volume 1, (Notes by N.D. Fowkes), Mathematical Association of America, 1966.

> The mousetrap chain reaction model was developed by Carrier for a course on mathematical modeling taught at Harvard University. In its original form, it was assumed that each mousetrap launched k = 2 ping-pong balls.

Maki, D.P. and M. Thompson, Mathematical Models and Applications, Prentice-Hall, Englewood Cliffs, N.J., 1973.

> In section 9.2 the model for the spread of a rumor is treated in detail. This presentation was used in the preparation of these notes.

Chapter 3. Stochastic Epidemic Models

In this section we consider the stochastic versions of the three deterministic models treated earlier. By virtue of the substantially increased difficulty of the mathematics involved, only the first model will be analysed in detail. The latter two models require techniques which are beyond the scope of the present treatment.

It is convenient to begin by restating the assumptions which are common to all of the models, both deterministic and stochastic:

      a.   The disease is transmitted by contact between an infected individual and a susceptible individual.

      b.   There is no latent period for the disease, hence the disease is transmitted instantaneously upon contact.

      c.   All susceptible individuals are equally susceptible and all infected individuals are equally infectious.

      d.   The population under consideration is fixed in size. This means that no birth or migration occurs, and all deaths are taken into account.

I.   The Trivial Model   (Yule-Furry or Pure Birth Process)

Consider a population which is effectively infinite in size. Initially everyone in the population is susceptible to the disease with the exception of one individual who is already infected.

Let the independent variable be time, t, and let:

$$I(t) = \text{Number of infected individuals at time } t$$

n.b. $I(t)$ is an integer valued random variable. Consequently, we will not be able to find $I(t)$ itself, but rather the probability that $I(t) = i : i = 1, 2, 3, \ldots$ as a function of time. Hence we define

$$p_i(t) = \text{Prob}\{I(t) = i\}$$

Notice that the single integer valued random variable $I(t)$ is described by an infinite family of probability density functions $p_i(t) : i = 1, 2, 3, \ldots$.

Also let

$\lambda\Delta t = $ Probability of a contact between a susceptible person and a particular infective which leads to a new case of the disease in the small interval of time Δt.

n.b. λ, which is called the infection rate, play the role that B played in the deterministic version of the same model. It is a parameter which can be used to fit the model to experimental data.

We would now like to determine $p_i(t+\Delta t)$, assuming that Δt is so small that at most one new case of the disease can arise in the interval from t to t+Δt. Recognize that two mutually exclusive situations can lead to this:

1.   At time t, there are i-1 infectives in the population with probability $p_{i-1}(t)$, and one of the i-1 infectives transmits the disease to a susceptible with probability $(i-1)\lambda\Delta t$.

2.   At time t, there are i infectives in the population with probability $p_i(t)$, and none of the i infectives transmits the disease to a susceptible with probability $(1-i\lambda\Delta t)$.

n.b.   More precisely, the expression for none of the i infectives transmitting the disease is:

$$(1 - \lambda\Delta t)^i = 1 - i\lambda\Delta t + o(\Delta t) \approx 1 - i\lambda\Delta t$$

where the notation $o(\cdot)$ has the following meaning:

If $f(x) \to 0$ as $x \to 0$ then $f(x)$ is $o(1)$
If $f(x)/x \to 0$ as $x \to 0$ then $f(x)$ is $o(x)$, etc.

It therefore follows that

$$p_i(t+\Delta t) = p_{i-1}(t) \cdot (i-1)\lambda\Delta t + p_i(t) \cdot (1 - i\lambda\Delta t)$$

Next, rearrange and let $\Delta t \to 0$ to yield

$$\frac{d}{dt} p_i(t) = -\lambda i p_i(t) + \lambda(i-1)p_{i-1}(t)$$

This is called a Differential-Difference Equation. Its solution tells
the probability that the population contains exactly i infectives at
time t, for all values of i. As with any differential equation of the
first order, it requires one initial condition. This condition
follows from the observation that at time t=0, the population contains
one infective, hence:

$$p_1(0) = 1$$

thus
$$p_i(0) = 0 \; ; \; i = 2, 3, 4, \ldots$$

Note further that since the number of infectives can only increase
as time passes, $p_0(t) = 0$ for all t.

Before looking into methods of solution, we restate the problem in
simplified notation, using $d(\cdot)/dt = (\cdot)'$ and $p_i(t) = p_i$:

$$p_i' = -\lambda i p_i + \lambda(i-1)p_{i-1} \; : \; p_1(0)=1, \; p_i(0)=0, \; i \neq 1$$

Methods of Solution: We proceed now to survey a number of the
different techniques which are available for solving Differential-
Difference Equations. The first and most direct of these consists of
solving the equations sequentially for increasing values of i, and
then using induction on i.

Notice that if we set i=1 in the general Differential-Difference
Equation, we find:

$$p_1' = -\lambda p_1 \; : \; p_1(0) = 1$$

This equation can be separated and integrated. The result is

$$p_1(t) = \exp\{-\lambda t\}$$

Next, set i=2 in the general Differential-Difference Equation to get

$$p_2' = -2\lambda p_2 + \lambda p_1 \; : \; p_2(0) = 0$$

However, we know the form of p_1 from the calculation above, so

$$p_2' + 2\lambda p_2 = \lambda \exp\{-\lambda t\}$$

Identify this as a first order, non-homogeneous differential equation.
Observe that if we multiply both sides by $\exp\{2\lambda t\}$ (called an
integrating factor), the resulting equation can be integrated directly
since the left hand side is the derivative of a product:

$$d[p_2 \exp\{2\lambda t\}] = \lambda \exp\{\lambda t\}$$

Multiplying through by dt and integrating formally leads to

$$p_2 \exp\{2\lambda t\} = \exp\{\lambda t\} + \text{constant}$$

The constant of integration is evaluated using the fact that $p_2(0) = 0$; hence the constant is -1, and the solution is

$$p_2(t) = \exp\{-\lambda t\}[1 - \exp\{-\lambda t\}]$$

Next, set i=3 in the general Differential-Difference Equation to get

$$p_3' + 3\ p_3 = 2\lambda\exp\{-\lambda t\}[1 - \exp\{-\lambda t\}]^2$$

But this can be integrated directly using the integrating factor $\exp\{3\lambda t\}$; the result is:

$$p_3(t) = \exp\{-\lambda t\}[1 - \exp\{-\lambda t\}]^2$$

We could continue in this manner, though the pattern should by now be apparent. It follows by induction that the general term is

$$p_i(t) = \exp\{-\lambda t\}[1 - \exp\{-\lambda t\}]^{i-1}$$

So now we know $p_i(t)$. But what we really want to know is the expected number of infectives in the population as a function of time. We must therefore evaluate:

$$E[I(t)] = \sum_{i=1}^{\infty} ip_i(t)$$

To save a bit of writing, let $z = \exp\{-\lambda t\}$, so that $p_i(t) = z(1-z)^{i-1}$, and

$$E[I(t)] = z \sum_{i=1}^{\infty} i(1-z)^{i-1} = -z \frac{d}{dz} \sum_{i=1}^{\infty} (1-z)^i$$

$$= -z \frac{d}{dz}(1/z) = 1/z = \exp\{\lambda t\}$$

Recall that the result for the deterministic version of this model was

$$I(t) = I_o \exp\{Bt\}$$

hence, with $I_o = 1$ and $B = \lambda$, the expected number of infectives in the stochastic version is identical to the number of infectives in the deterministic version.

n.b. It is not hard to show that if the initial number of infectives in the stochastic model is taken to be I_o, then $E[I(t)] = I_o \exp\{\lambda t\}$ as one would expect.

It is also a simple matter to work out the variance in the number of infectives as a function of time.

$$V[I(t)] = E[I(t)^2] - E[I(t)]^2$$

$$= \sum_{i=1}^{\infty} i^2 p_i(t) - \exp\{2\lambda t\}$$

$$\rightarrow \quad V[I(t)] = \exp\{\lambda t\}[\exp\{\lambda t\} - 1]$$

Notice that the variance grows without bound as time passes; however, the coefficient of variation, C.V., remains bounded as $t \rightarrow \infty$:

$$C.V. = \frac{\sqrt{V[I(t)]}}{E[I(t)]} = \sqrt{1 - \exp\{-\lambda t\}} \rightarrow 1 \text{ as } t \rightarrow \infty$$

This suggests that the deterministic version of the model provides a useful approximation to the actual answer. Unfortunately, as was noted earlier, the deterministic solution is unrealistic in that it leads to unbounded growth, due to a basic fault in the model.

We proceed now to investigate several other possible methods of solution.

The next method we investigate is solution by means of Laplace Transformations. The idea is to apply a particular operation to each term in the Differential-Difference Equation so as to transform the equation into an algebraic expression without any derivatives. The equation is then solved, and the result is transformed back into the original variables. Although in general the mathematics needed to invert the transformed solution is beyond the scope of this treatment, certain tricks can be employed to find the answer.

n.b. If this description sounds mysterious, consider the following analogy. Imagine that you wish to evaluate

$$x = [27]^{1/3}$$

Since no procedure exists for evaluating fractional powers, apply the transformation "logarithm" to both sides to get:

$$\ell n \ x = \ell n[27]^{1/3} = \frac{1}{3} \ell n \ 27 = \frac{3.2958}{3} = 1.0986$$

The solution is now found by applying the proper inversion operation. In this case it is of course "exponentiation"; however, even if one did not know that fact, the answer could be found by consulting a table of natural logarithms and looking up 1.0986 to learn that $x = 3$.

The Laplace Transformation of $p_i(t)$ is defined by the operation:

$$L[p_i(t)] \equiv \int_0^\infty \exp\{-st\} \ p_i(t) \ dt \equiv P_i(s)$$

Consequently, the Laplace Transformation of the derivative is:

$$L[p_i'(t)] = \int_0^\infty \exp\{-st\}p_i'(t)\ dt$$

(integrate by parts)
$$= \exp\{-st\}p_i(t)\ \Big|_0^\infty + s \int_0^\infty \exp\{-st\}p_i(t)\ dt$$

$$= -p_i(0) + sP_i(s)$$

Laplace Transforming both sides of the Differential-Difference Equation then leads to:

$$sP_i(s) = -\lambda i P_i(s) + \lambda(i-1)P_{i-1}(s) \quad : i = 2,\ 3,\ 4,\ldots$$

and when $i = 1$:

$$-1 + sP_1(s) = -\lambda P_1(s)$$

Thus

$$P_i(s) = \frac{\lambda(i-1)}{s + \lambda i} P_{i-1}(s) \quad : i = 2,\ 3,\ 4,\ \ldots$$

and

$$P_1(s) = \frac{1}{s + \lambda}$$

Identify this as a linear Difference Equation which is in fact a form which submits immediately to iterative solution. The result is

$$P_i(s) = \frac{(i-1)\lambda}{s + i\lambda} P_{i-1}(s)$$

$$= \frac{(i-1)\lambda}{s + i\lambda} \cdot \frac{(i-2)\lambda}{s + (i-1)\lambda} P_{i-2}(s)$$

$$\vdots$$

$$= \frac{(i-1)\lambda}{s + i\lambda} \cdot \frac{(i-2)\lambda}{s + (i-1)\lambda} \cdot \cdot \cdot \frac{\lambda}{s + 2\lambda} \cdot P_1(s)$$

$$= \frac{(i-1)!\ \lambda^{i-1}}{(s+i\lambda)\cdots(s+\lambda)}$$

We must now deduce how to invert this expression to get back $p_i(t)$. Perhaps the easiest way is to observe that

$$L[\exp\{-i\lambda t\}] = \frac{1}{s + i\lambda}$$

thus

$$L^{-1}[1/(s+i\lambda)] = \exp\{-i\lambda t\}$$

It therefore follows immediately that

$$p_1(t) = L^{-1}[P_1(s)] = L^{-1}[1/(s+\lambda)] = \exp\{-\lambda t\}$$

Next, look at the inversion of $P_2(s)$. By employing partial fractions, it follows easily that

$$P_2(t) = L^{-1}[1/(s+\lambda)] - L^{-1}[1/(s+2\lambda)]$$

$$= \exp\{-\lambda t\} - \exp\{-2\lambda t\}$$

Proceeding in this manner, and then using induction leads to:

$$P_i(t) = \sum_{j=0}^{i-1} \binom{i-1}{j} (-1)^j \exp\{-(j-1)\lambda t\}$$

$$= \exp\{-\lambda t\}[1 - \exp\{-\lambda t\}]^{i-1}$$

n.b. This is of course the same result as before. The utility of the Laplace Transformation is not immediately obvious here; however, for some complicated stochastic processes, this method succeeds while the more direct one fails.

At this point we might well ask why we bother to find $p_i(t)$ when in fact we are really interested in the moments (expectation, variance, etc.) of the random variable, $I(t)$. The answer is that we often also wish to know $p_i(t)$. However, for those occasions when the moments are sufficient, some other techniques are available. We proceed now to consider some of these techniques.

To calculate the expected number of infectives in the population as a function of time directly, proceed as follows. Start with the definition of the expectation:

$$E[I(t)] \equiv E = \sum_{i=1}^{\infty} i\, p_i$$

Notice immediately that since $p_1(0) - 1$ and $p_i(0) = 0 : i - 2, 3, \ldots$

$$E(0) = 1$$

Next, differentiate the definition of the expectation with respect to time to get:

$$E' = \sum_{i=1}^{\infty} i\, p_i'$$

where, as before, prime denotes differentiation with respect to time.

Next, use the Differential-Difference Equation to replace p_i':

$$E' = \sum_{i=1}^{\infty} i\,[-\lambda i p_i + \lambda(i-1)p_{i-1}]$$

$$= \lambda \sum_{k=1}^{\infty} [-k^2 + (k+1)k]\,p_k = \lambda \sum_{k=1}^{\infty} k\,p_k$$

Thus, from the definition of the expectation:

$$E' = \lambda E \qquad : E(0) = 1$$

This is a simple Differential Equation which can be separated and integrated directly to yield:

$$E \equiv E[I(t)] = \exp\{\lambda t\}$$

One can continue in this manner to find the variance $V[I(t)]$, and in fact, as many higher moments as one cares to work out.

A more sophisticated version of this method is also available. The advantage of this method is that it finds all of the moments simultaneously. There is also a disadvantage, and that is that we must solve a Partial Differential Equation.

We begin by defining the Moment Generating Function, $M(\theta,t)$:

$$M(\theta,t) = \sum_{i=1}^{\infty} \exp\{i\theta\}p_i(t) = E[\exp\{I(t)\theta\}]$$

By formal manipulation, it then follows that:

$$\frac{\partial M(\theta,t)}{\partial t} = \sum_{i=1}^{\infty} \exp\{i\theta\}\,p_i'$$

$$\frac{\partial M(\theta,t)}{\partial \theta} = \sum_{i=1}^{\infty} i\,\exp\{i\theta\}p_i$$

By multiplying the Differential-Difference Equation through by $\exp\{i\theta\}$ and summing from $i=1$ to $i=\infty$, it follows immediately that

$$\sum_{i=1}^{\infty} \exp\{i\theta\}\,p_i' = -\lambda \sum_{i=1}^{\infty} i\,\exp\{i\theta\}p_i + \lambda \sum_{i=1}^{\infty} (i-1)\exp\{i\theta\}p_{i-1}$$

Hence, from the definitions above:

$$\frac{\partial M}{\partial t} = \lambda[\exp\{\theta\} - 1]\frac{\partial M}{\partial \theta}$$

Identify this as a Partial Differential Equation of the first order. The appropriate side condition follows from the fact that $p_1(0) = 1$, $p_i(0) = 0$: $i = 2, 3, \ldots$, which leads to:

$$M(\theta,0) = \exp\{\theta\}$$

n.b. Partial Differential Equations of the first order can be solved by a method due to LaGrange. This method is outlined in the Appendix to this chapter.

The subsidiary equation is given by:

$$\frac{dt}{1} = \frac{d\theta}{-\lambda[\exp\{\theta\} - 1]} = \frac{dM}{0}$$

The equality between the first and third terms tells us that:

$$u(M,\theta,t) = M = \text{constant}$$

and the equality between the first and second terms tells us that:

$$dt = \frac{\exp\{-\theta\}\,d\theta}{-\lambda[1-\exp\{-\theta\}]}$$

This can be integrated directly to yield:

$$t = -\frac{1}{\lambda}\ln[1 - \exp\{-\theta\}] + \text{constant}$$

This last expression can be rearranged into the form:

$$v(m,\theta,t) = \exp\{\lambda t\}(1 - \exp\{-\theta\}) = \text{constant}$$

It therefore follows that:

$$M(\theta,t) = \Psi[\exp\{\lambda t\}(1 - \exp\{-\theta\})]$$

We now appeal to the side condition $M(\theta,0) = \exp\{\theta\}$, which tells us:

$$M(\theta,0) = \Psi[1 - \exp\{-\theta\}] = \exp\{\theta\}$$

Let $w = 1 - \exp\{-\theta\}$ $\rightarrow$ $\exp\{\theta\} = 1/(1-w)$, hence:

$$\Psi[w] = 1/(1-w)$$

n.b. This expression tells us the explicit form of the function $\Psi[\cdot]$, which is the solution we seek.

Thus, $$M(\theta,t) = \Psi[\exp\{\lambda t\}(1 - \exp\{-\theta\})]$$

$$= [1 - \exp\{\lambda t\}(1 - \exp\{-\theta\})]^{-1}$$

To complete the illustration, we now derive $E[I(t)]$ from $M(\theta,t)$.
Since

$$M(\theta,t) = E[\exp\{I(t)\theta\}]$$

it follows that

$$E[I(t)] = \left.\frac{\partial M}{\partial \theta}\right|_{\theta=0}$$

$$= \left.\frac{\partial}{\partial \theta}[1 - \exp\{\lambda t\}(1 - \exp\{-\theta\})]^{-1}\right|_{\theta=0}$$

$$= \left.\frac{\exp\{\lambda t\}}{1 - \exp\{\lambda t\}(1 - \exp\{-\theta\})^2}\right|_{\theta=0}$$

$$= \exp\{\lambda t\}$$

Higher moments are easily found by manipulating the Moment Generating Function.

n.b. An exactly analogous procedure employing the Probability Generating Function:

$$P(s,t) = \sum_{i=1}^{\infty} s^i p_i(t) = E[s^{I(t)}]$$

leads to a Partial Differential Equation whose solution yields the $p_i(t)$.

II. The Stochastic Simple Epidemic Model

As with the deterministic version, the stochastic trivial model is defective in that it treats the pool of susceptibles as infinite in size. To improve the model, we assume that the population under consideration numbers N individuals at all times. Further, at the start there is just one infective and so there are $N-1$ susceptibles.

In addition to the variables defined for the trivial model, let

S(t) = Number of susceptibles at time t.

n.b. We must now keep track of two integer valued random variables, I(t) and S(t). This would suggest that we introduce a joint density function

$$p_{ij}(t) = \text{Prob}\{I(t) = i, S(t) = j\}$$

However, since we know that $I(t) + S(t) = N$, we can continue to work with our old density, redefined as follows:

$$p_i(t) = \text{Prob } \{I(t) = i, \ S(t) = N - i\}$$

We also need to define a probabilistic contact rate constant:

$\beta \Delta t$ = Probability of a contact between a particular susceptible and a particular infective which leads to a new case of the disease in the small interval of time Δt.

Instead of deriving the Differential-Difference Equation for the stochastic process from first principles, we generalize the equation for the trivial model. Recall that this equation was:

$$p_i' = -\lambda i p_i + \lambda(i-1)p_{i-1}$$

The coefficient λi represented the situation in which none of the i infectives transmitted the disease. This generalizes to $\beta i(N-i)$, representing the situation where none of the i infectives transmits the disease to one of the N-i susceptibles. Similarly, the coefficient $\lambda(i-1)$ represented the situation in which exactly one of the i-1 infectives transmitted the disease. This generalizes to $\beta(i-1)(N-i+1)$, representing the situation where exactly one of the i-1 infectives transmits the disease to one of the N-(i-1) susceptibles. The Differential-Difference Equation is therefore of the form:

$$p_i' = -\beta i(N-i)p_i + \beta(i-1)(N-i+1)p_{i-1}$$

n.b. Although this equation is almost identical in form to the one for the trivial model, it is now nonlinear in the index i. This fact causes considerable difficulty. In fact, it does not appear to be possible to write down a simple, closed-form expression for either the $p_i(t)$ or for the moments.

For this reason, it is unproductive to continue our analysis any further. All methods at our disposal lead to disappointingly messy and uninformative expressions. There is, however, one interesting question which we can answer without undue complication. Specifically, is the expected value of I(t) for the stochastic model the same as the solution to the deterministic analog?

To answer this question, we first recall the governing equation for the deterministic model:

$$\frac{dI(t)}{dt} = \beta I(t)[N - I(t)] \quad : \quad I(0) = 1$$

It therefore follows directly that

$$\left.\frac{dI}{dt}\right|_{t=0} = \beta(N-1)$$

and by differentiating once

$$\left.\frac{d^2I}{dt^2}\right|_{t=0} = \beta\left(N\frac{dI}{dt} - 2I\frac{dI}{dt}\right)_{t=0} = \beta^2(N-2)(N-1)$$

We now compare these values with the corresponding ones for the stochastic version of the model. Start with the definition of the expectation

$$E[I(t)] = \sum_{i=1}^{N} ip_i(t) \qquad : p_1(0) = 1$$

Thus

$$E[I(0)] = 1$$

as with the deterministic model. Next, differentiate the definition of the expectation, make use of the Differential-Difference Equation, and evaluate at t=0 to get:

$$\left.\frac{dE[I]}{dt}\right|_{t=0} = \sum_{i=1}^{N} ip_i'(0)$$

$$= \sum_{i=1}^{N} i\{-\beta i(N-i)p_i(0) + \beta(i-1)(N-i+1)p_{i-1}(0)\}$$

$$= -\beta(N-1) + 2\beta(N-1) = \beta(N-1)$$

as with the deterministic model. Finally, differentiate the definition of the expectation a second time, make use of the Differential-Difference Equation, and evaluate at t=0 to get:

$$\left.\frac{d^2E[I]}{dt^2}\right|_{t=0} = \sum_{i=1}^{N} ip_i''(0) + \beta^2(N-3)(N-1)$$

which is different than the result for the deterministic version of the model.

The answer to our question therefore is that the expected value of I(t) as found from the stochastic formulation is not the same as the result for the analogous deterministic model. It is however the case that the larger the value of N, the more nearly coincident the results become.

Typical epidemic curves for small N are sketched below.

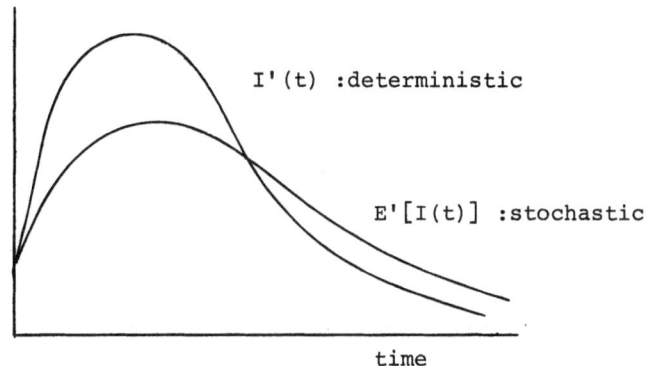

I'(t) :deterministic

E'[I(t)] :stochastic

time

III.   The Stochastic General Epidemic Model

The stochastic version of the general epidemic model follows by
including the possibility of removal of infectives from circulation.

In addition to the variables employed for the simple stochastic model
we need to introduce:

$R(t)$ = Number of removed individuals at time t.

$\gamma \Delta t$ = Probability that a particular infective will be
removed from circulation during the short time
interval Δt.

$S(t)$, $I(t)$ and $R(t)$ are now all integer valued random variables which
satisfy $S(t) + I(t) + R(t) = N$. Consequently, we must now introduce a
joint density function of the form:

$$P_{i,r}(t) = \text{Prob} \{I(t) = i, \quad R(t) = r, \quad \& \quad S(t) = N-i-r \}$$

If we make the usual assumption that only one "event" (infection or
removal) can occur during a short interval of time, then there are
just three possibilities:

1.   A susceptible becomes infected: (s+1, i-1, r) → (s, i, r)

2.   An infective becomes removed: (s, i+1, r-1) → (s, i, r)

3.   Neither of the above transitions occurs: (s, i, r) → (s, i, r)

By analogy with our earlier development, this leads to the equation:

$$P'_{i,r} = -[\beta i (N-i-r) + \gamma i] P_{i,r} + \beta (i-1)(N-i-r+1) P_{i-1,r} + \gamma (i+1) P_{i+1,r-1}$$

since this equation cannot be solved, we proceed no further.

Appendix   LaGrange's Method:

Suppose we wish to solve the linear Partial Differential Equation:

$$P(x,y,z) \frac{\partial z}{\partial x} + Q(x,y,z) \frac{\partial z}{\partial y} = R(x,y,z)$$

subject to some appropriate side condition(s). First, form the subsidiary equation in the form:

$$\frac{dx}{P} = \frac{dy}{Q} = \frac{dz}{R}$$

Next, find two independent integrals of these equations by considering the equalities pair-wise. Write these in the form

$$u(x,y,z) = \text{constant}$$
$$v(x,y,z) = \text{constant}$$

The most general solution of the Partial Differential Equation is then given by:

$$u = \Psi(v)$$

where Ψ is an arbitrary function. Surprisingly, the form of this function can be found by an appeal to the side condition(s).

n.b. For the problem treated in these notes:

$$x = t, \qquad y = \theta, \qquad z = M$$
$$P = 1, \qquad Q = -\lambda(\exp\{\theta\}-1), \qquad R = 0$$

Problems

1. If an epidemic is described by a Pure Birth Process:

$$\frac{d}{dt} p_i(t) = -\lambda i p_i(t) + \lambda(i-1)p_{i-1}(t)$$

and the initial number of infectives is $I(0) = m$, verify by induction using the Differential-Difference Equation that

$$p_i(t) = \binom{i-1}{m-1} \exp\{-m\lambda t\}[1 - \exp\{-\lambda t\}]^{i-m} \quad : i = m, \; m+1, \; \ldots$$

2. For the epidemic described in problem 1, find $E[I(t)]$ and $V[I(t)]$.

3. Given that

$$P_3(s) = \frac{2\lambda^2}{(s+3\lambda)\,(s+2\lambda)\,(s+\lambda)}$$

is the Laplace Transform of $p_3(t)$, employ partial fractions to evaluate $p_3(t)$.

4. Solve the Differential-Difference Equation for the Pure Birth
    Process as given in problem 1 directly for the variance $V[I(t)]$,
    assuming that the initial number of infectives $I(0) = 1$.

    Hint: Use $V(X) = E(X^2) - \overline{E(X)}^2$

5. Make use of the definition of the Probability Generating Function:

$$P(s,t) = \sum_{i=1}^{\infty} s^i p_i(t) \quad = E[s^{I(t)}]$$

    to transform the Differential-Difference Equation for the Pure
    Birth Process as given in problem 1 above into a Partial
    Differential Equation. Then apply LaGrange's Method to find the
    solution for the case $I(0) = 1$.

6. Show that for the stochastic simple epidemic model, in which

$$p_i' = -\beta i(N-i)p_i + \beta(i-1)(N-i+1)p_{i-1} \quad : p_1(0) = 1$$

    the quantity $E''[I(0)] = \beta^2(N-3)(N-1)$

References

The material in this section can be found in virtually any text on
mathematical epidemiology, as well as in a number of books on
mathematical modeling. Some useful books are:

Bailey, N.T.J., The Mathematical Theory of Infectious Diseases,
        Hafner Press, New York, 1975.

        This is perhaps the most comprehensive book on the subject of
        mathematical epidemiology. The second and third models in
        these notes are discussed in detail in sections 5.3 -5.5 and
        6.3 respectively.

Bailey, N.T.J., The Elements of Stochastic Processes, John Wiley and
        Sons, New York, 1964.

        The pure birth process is discussed in section 8.1 - 8.2.
        The method of LaGrange is described in section 7.5. The
        remainder of the book provides many useful discussions of
        other types of stochastic processes.

Ludwig, D., Stochastic Population Theories, Lecture Notes in
        Biomathematics Volume 3, Springer-Verlag, New York, 1974.

The first and second models are treated in sections I.2.1 and I.2.3 respectively. The third model is treated in detail in section II.2.0 and II.2.1 (Advanced).

Maki, D.P. and M. Thompson, Mathematical Models and Applications, Prentice-Hall, Englewood Cliffs, N.J., 1973.

The technique for showing that the deterministic and stochastic simple epidemic models lead to different results is taken from section 9.1 of this book.

Chapter 4. Chain Binomial Models

We look next at both the deterministic and stochastic versions of the chain binomial model. Although this model was originally designed as an educational device, it has proven to be a useful representation for analysing small epidemics, such as those within a single family or a school.

The central idea of the model is that the disease possesses a fixed length latent period which is used as one unit of model time. The period of infectiousness is then contracted to a point in time, and indexed by n = 0, 1, 2, ...

n.b. This is strongly reminiscent of the mousetrap chain reaction, with the flight time of the ping-pong balls corresponding with the latent period, and the springing of the traps corresponding with the infectious period (instant).

As usual, we recognize three classes of individuals; susceptibles, infectives, and removals, denoted by S_n, I_n, and R_n, respectively.

Further, the disease is assumed to render the removals immune, hence the natural progression susceptible to infective to removed occurs. Also, the total population is fixed at all times at N, so

$$S_n + I_n + R_n = N$$

and the infectives remain infected for one unit of model time and then automatically are removals.

n.b. This too is effectively identical to the mousetrap chain reaction.

What is new is the manner in which the disease is transmitted. Imagine that just prior to an infectious period there are S_n susceptibles and I_n infectives. Consider one particular susceptible, assuming always that the probability of sufficient contact between any one infective and any one susceptible to cause infection is p. Hence the probability of no transmission on a pair-wise contact between a susceptible and an infective is $q = 1 - p$. But to avoid catching the disease, the susceptible under scrutiny must avoid sufficient contact with each of the I_n infectives independently, thus

$$Q_n = (1 - p)^{I_n} = q^{I_n}$$

where Q_n is the probability of a particular susceptible avoiding infection during one time interval when there are I_n infectives.

The probability that there are no infectives at time n+1 is then:

$$\text{Prob}\{S_{n+1} = S_n, \; I_{n+1} = 0 \mid S_n, \; I_n\} = Q_n^{S_n}$$

The probability of exactly one infective at time n+1 is similarly:

$$\text{Prob}\{S_{n+1} = S_n - 1, \; I_{n+1} = 1 \mid S_n, \; I_n\} = \binom{S_n}{1} Q_n^{S_n - 1} (1 - Q_n)$$

In general, the probability of exactly I infectives at time n+1, given that there were S_n susceptibles and I_n infectives at time n, is:

$$\text{Prob}\{S_{n+1} = S_n - I, \; I_{n+1} = I \mid S_n, \; I_n\} = \binom{S_n}{I} Q_n^{S_n - I} (1 - Q_n)^{I}$$

Assuming that we know q, S_n, and I_n, we can easily find the expected number of susceptibles and infectives at time n+1:

$$E\{I_{n+1} \mid S_n, \; I_n\} = \sum_{I=0}^{S_n} I \; \text{Prob}\{S_{n+1} = S_n - I, \; I_{n+1} = I \mid S_n, \; I_n\}$$

$$= \sum_{I=0}^{S_n} I \binom{S_n}{I} Q_n^{S_n - I} (1 - Q_n)^{I} = S_n (1 - Q_n)$$

$$E\{S_{n+1} \mid S_n, \; I_n\} = S_n - E\{I_{n+1} \mid S_n, \; I_n\} = S_n Q_n$$

Of course what we would really like to know are the unconditional expectations, which depend only upon q, S_0 and I_0. Before looking more carefully at removing the conditioning on the state of the

epidemic at the previous time interval, we investigate the
deterministic analog of the chain binomial model.

n.b. For notational convenience, we introduce the following variable
  analogies:

$$S_n \to s_n, \quad I_n \to i_n, \quad \text{and } R_n \to r_n$$

  where the lower case letters are the deterministic equivalents of
  the integer valued random variables denoted by the capitals.

As with the stochastic model, the fraction of pair-wise contacts
between a particular susceptible and particular infective which lead
to infection is denoted by p, hence a fraction $q = 1 - p$ do not lead to
infection.

In each successive time interval, the available susceptibles from the
prior time interval are split into two groups, one group still
susceptible, the other infected, thus:

$$s_n = s_{n+1} + i_{n+1}$$

This division depends upon the number of infectives at time n in the
following manner. The fraction which remains uninfected avoid contact
with all infectives, hence:

$$q_n = q^{i_n}$$

and the remainder, $1 - q_n$, become infected.

This leads to the following expressions for the number of susceptibles
and infectives at time n+1:

$$s_{n+1} = s_n q_n$$

$$i_{n+1} = s_n (1 - q_n)$$

These we identify as Difference Equations. Given the initial
conditions s_0 and i_0, it then follows that:

$$s_1 = s_0 q_0 = s_0 q^{i_0}$$

$$s_2 = s_1 q_1 = s_0 q_0 q_1 = s_0 q^{i_0 + i_1}$$

and by induction:

$$s_{n+1} = s_0 q^{\sum_{j=0}^{n} i_j}$$

However, since the total number of individuals at risk of contracting

44

the disease is fixed at N, as $n \to \infty$, $i \to 0$, and $s_n \to s_\infty$, the number of ussceptibles remaining after the epidemic is over. Thus:

$$s_\infty = s_0 q^{N-s_\infty}$$

Next, define $\sigma_0 = s_0/N$, $\sigma_\infty = s_\infty/N$, and $k = -N \ln q > 0$ to get:

$$\sigma_\infty = \sigma_0 \exp\{-k(1 - \sigma_\infty)\}$$

To understand the possible outcomes of an epidemic, we·study this expression graphically. Imagine for a moment that $\sigma_0 = 1$. In the figure below, two possible functions from the right hand side are plotted, one with $k>1$, the other with $k<1$. The solution corresponds with the intersection of the curved lines with the straight line.

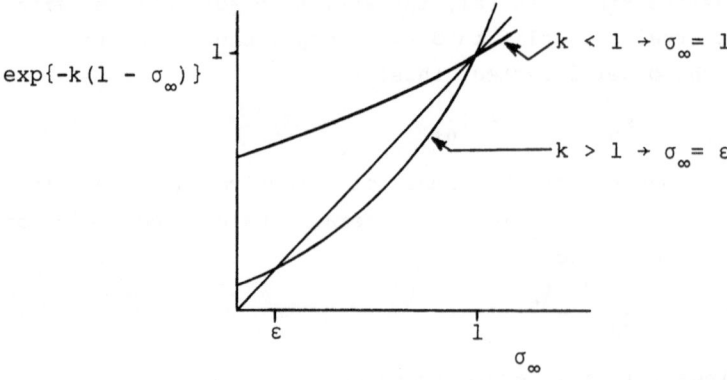

n.b. To decide which curve corresponds with $k>1$, simply note that the slope of the exponential curve at $\sigma_\infty = 1$ is k.

In actuality, $\sigma_0 < 1$, though ordinarily not by much. The figure below is drawn for a realistic value of σ_0:

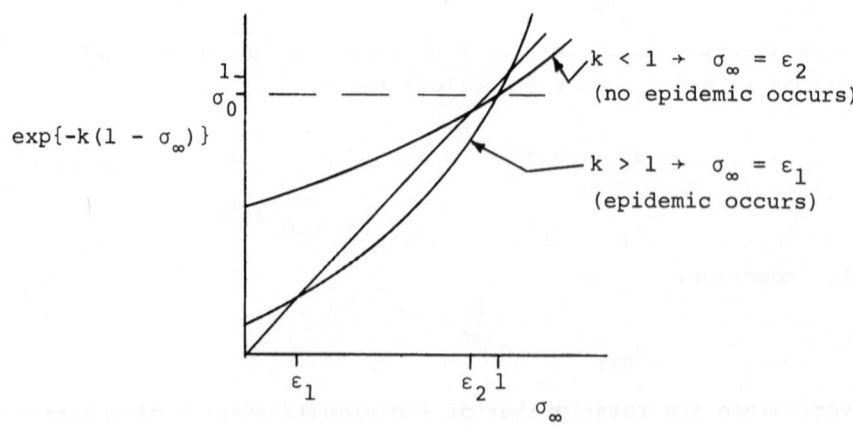

We therefore conclude that the deterministic version of the chain
binomial model exhibits a threshold behavior depending upon whether
$k<1$ or $k>1$.

We return now to the stochastic version. Recall that the expected
number of susceptibles was given by the relation:

$$E\{S_{n+1}|S_n, I_n\} = S_n q^{I_n}$$

Hence, if we know q, S_0, and I_0, it follows that

$$E\{S_1\} = S_0 q^{I_0}$$

n.b. This is an unconditional expectation since S_0 and I_0 are known
     deterministically.

Next, we find that

$$E\{S_2|S_1, I_1\} = S_1 q^{I_1}$$

where $I_1 + S_1 = S_0$. Thus

$$E\{S_2|I_1\} = (S_0 - I_1)q^{I_1}$$

and the unconditional expectation is therefore:

$$E\{S_2\} = E[E\{S_2|I_1\}] = E\{(S_0 - I_1)q^{I_1}\}$$

$$= \sum_{I_1=0}^{S_0} (S_0 - I_1)q^{I_1} \binom{S_0}{I_1} Q_0^{S_0-I_1}(1 - Q_0)^{I_1}$$

$$\rightarrow \quad = S_0 q^{I_0}[q + (1 - q) q^{I_0}]^{S_0-1}$$

n.b. In working out this result, we have made use of the fact that:

$$\sum_{j=0}^{N} s^j \binom{N}{j} p^j (1 - p)^{N-j} = (1 - p + sp)^N$$

If the result for $E\{S_2\}$ is compared with the deterministic analog:

$$s_2 = s_0 q^{i_0+ i_1} \quad : \quad i_1 = s_0 - s_1 = s_0[1 - q^{i_0}]$$

for the values: $S_0 = s_0 = 10$, $I_0 = i_0 = 1$, $q = 0.9$, it follows easily that:

$$E\{S_2\} = 9[.99]^9 \approx 8.22$$

$$i_1 = 10(1 - .9) = 1, \quad s_2 = 10[.9]^2 = 8.1 \neq 8.22$$

n.b. It is interesting to note that if in the stochastic model we let

$$E\{S_{n+1}|S_n, I_n\} \quad \rightarrow \quad E\{S_{n+1}|\bar{S}_n, \bar{I}_n\}$$

where $\quad \bar{S}_n = E\{S_n\} \quad$ and $\quad \bar{I}_n = E\{I_n\}$

as we did with the mousetrap model, the stochastic result becomes identical with the deterministic result. This of course means that we have discarded an interesting aspect of the stochastic solution since the deterministic and stochastic formulations do not yield the same results.

We have reached something of an impasse. We have rejected the deterministic version of the model as inadequate for predicting the results of the stochastic model. However, we are unable to continue in an acceptably simple mathematical manner. Let us illustrate the problem. We have worked out the unconditional expectation $E\{S_2\}$ and could with a similar amount of work find $E\{I_2\}$ directly. We could then calculate:

$$E\{S_3|S_2, I_2\} \quad \text{and} \quad E\{I_3|S_2, I_2\}$$

and then get rid of the conditioning using $E\{S_2\}$ and $E\{I_2\}$. We could do this repeatedly to find successive unconditional expectations of S_n and I_n. However, each successive calculation becomes more complicated than the one before. Although this is mechanical, it is not very interesting. We therefore look to other methods.

I. Direct Calculation

Assume that we are given n, q, S_0, and I_0. We then proceed to find

$$\text{Prob}\{S_1 = S_0 - I, \quad I_1 = I\} \quad : I = 0, 1, 2, \ldots, S_0$$

Next, for each pair of values (S_1, I_1), calculate:

$$\text{Prob}\{S_2 = S_1 - I, \quad I_2 = I | S_1, I_1\} \quad : I = 0, 1, 2, \ldots, S_1$$

and then the unconditional probabilities:

$$\text{Prob}\{S_2 = S_1 - I, \quad I_2 = I\} = \text{Prob}\{S_2 = S_1 - I, I_2 = I | S_1, I_1\} \cdot \text{Prob}\{S_1, I_1\}$$
$$: I = 0, 1, 2, \ldots, S_1$$

Keep going in this manner for a total of N steps.

·n.b. Clearly, since at each stage in the epidemic there must be at least one infective for the epidemic to continue, the epidemic must have ended after N steps.

Once the unconditional probabilities are known, it is a simple matter
to find the unconditional expectations:

$$E\{S_n\} = \sum_{S_n, I_n} S_n \cdot \text{Prob}\{S_n, I_n\}$$

$$E\{I_n\} = \sum_{S_n, I_n} I_n \cdot \text{Prob}\{S_n, I_n\}$$

While this method is attractive as it is easily implemented on a
computer, it has two major faults. First, it involves order(N^3)
calculations, and is therefore not practical for N greater than about
100. Second, if one wishes to adjust N, q, S_0, or I_0, one must go
back and recalculate all values.

II. Monte Carlo Simulation

Assume that we are given N, q, S_0 and I_0. Proceed to calculate

$$\text{Prob}\{S_1 = S_0 - I, \ I_1 = I\} \quad : \quad I = 0, 1, 2, \ldots, S_0$$

Use these probabilities (which of course sum to unity) to partition a
unit interval into $S_0 + 1$ pieces. Then generate a uniformly
distributed random number between 0 and 1. Its value determines I_1
and S_1. Proceed in this manner to simulate the epidemic many times,
and use statistical methods. The results not only provide expected
outcomes, they also demonstrate sample paths for the epidemic.

An attraction of this method is that it is easy to program, and for
each trial involves only order(N) calculations. Once again, there are
two major shortcomings. As with method I, any change in the
parameters requires complete recalculation. Also, it can be shown
that the error in the results only diminishes as $1/\sqrt{M}$, where M is the
number of trial runs. It therefore requires 100 times as many runs to
improve accuracy by one decimal place.

III. Backward Equations

Typically, data from an epidemic tells us how many people ultimately
contracted the disease. We therefore set out to calculate the final
size distribution directly. Assume that we are given N, q, S_0, and
I_0. What we will do is find:

$$P\{R_\infty | S_0\} = \text{Prob}\{\text{there are } R_\infty \text{ removals after epidemic } | S_0\}$$

We do this calculation constructively. Start off with $S_0 = 1$.

n.b. Recall that $Q_0 = q^{I_0}$ is the probability that a particular susceptible avoids contracting the disease during one infectious period from each of the I_0 infectives.

Clearly,

$$P\{0|1\} = Q_0 = q^{I_0}$$

$$P\{1|1\} = 1 - P\{0|1\} = 1 - Q_0$$

Next, consider $S_0 = 2$:

$$P\{0|2\} = Q_0^2$$

$$P\{1|2\} = 2P\{1|1\}Q_0 q$$

n.b. Let us dissect this expression: The term $P\{1|1\}$ represents the probability that one of the initial susceptibles ultimately gets the disease and is therefore removed. The term Q_0 represents the fact that the other initial susceptible does not get the disease from any of the initial infectives. The term q represents the fact that this same initial susceptible avoids getting the disease from the initial susceptible who becomes infected. The '2' results from the fact that this can occur in two exclusive ways.

Thus,

$$P\{2|2\} = 1 - P\{0|2\} - P\{1|2\}$$

Let us continue one more step before generalizing. Let $S_0 = 3$.

$$P\{0|3\} = Q_0^3$$

$$P\{1|3\} = 3P\{1|1\}Q_0^2 q^2$$

$$P\{2|3\} = 3P\{2|2\}Q_0 q^2$$

$$P\{3|3\} = 1 - P\{0|3\} - P\{1|3\} - P\{2|3\}$$

The procedure should by now be obvious.

For general S_0:

$$P\{0|S_0\} = Q_0^{S_0}$$

$$P\{R_\infty|S_0\} = \binom{S_0}{R_\infty} P\{R_\infty|R_\infty\}Q_0^{S_0-R_\infty} q^{R_\infty(S_0-R_\infty)} \quad : \quad S_0 > R_\infty$$

$$P\{S_0|S_0\} = 1 - \sum_{R_\infty=0}^{S_0-1} P\{R_\infty|S_0\}$$

The chief advantage to method III over the other two methods is that
one calculates the most interesting quantity concerning the epidemic
directly. Further, only about order(N^2) numbers are calculated.
The main disadvantages are that once again, one must start over if
any of the parameters change, and further, it turns out that the
$P\{R_\infty|R_\infty\}$ approach zero rapidly as $S_0 \to \infty$. The consequence is that the
method is imprecise for N greater than about 50.

It is worth noting that method III represents an ingenious way of
circumventing the really difficult part of the solution to the
stochastic chain binomial epidemic model. The inspiration for this
method was the observation that what one really wants to know is the
final size distribution after the epidemic, and not the state at every
step of the process. This idea of finding what is useful and
observeable should play a central role in all applied mathematics.

Appendix   Conditional Expectations

Although only the conditional expectation appeared in this chapter,
for the sake of completeness we include the conditional variance in
this appendix.

Let X and Y be two integer valued random variables which are not
independent, and imagine that we know the probability density function
for Y:

$$f_Y(y) = \text{Prob}\{Y = y\}$$

and the conditional probability density function for X given Y:

$$f_{X|Y}(x|y) = \text{Prob}\{X = x|Y = y\}$$

The marginal probability density function for X is then clearly

$$f_X(x) = \sum_y f_{X|Y}(x|y) \cdot f_Y(y) = \text{Prob}\{X = x\}$$

Example: Assume that we are told that Y is distributed according to a
Poisson density with parameter λ:

$$f_Y(y) = \frac{\lambda^y \exp\{-\lambda\}}{y!} \qquad : y = 0, 1, 2, \ldots$$

and the conditional density of X given Y is Binomially distributed with parameters y and ρ :

$$f_{X|Y}(x|y) = \binom{y}{x} \rho^x (1-\rho)^{y-x} \qquad : x = 0, 1, \ldots, y$$

It therefore follows that the marginal density for X is Poisson distributed with parameter $\lambda\rho$:

$$f_X(x) = \sum_{y=x}^{\infty} \binom{y}{x} \rho^x (1-\rho)^{y-x} \lambda^y \exp\{-\lambda\}/y!$$

$$= \frac{(\lambda\rho)^x \exp\{-\lambda\}}{x!} \sum_{y=x}^{\infty} \frac{1}{(y-x)!} [\lambda(1-\rho)]^{y-x}$$

$$= \frac{(\lambda\rho)^x \exp\{-\lambda\rho\}}{x!}$$

We next introduce the expectation which is defined:

$$E\{Y\} = \sum_y y\, f_Y(y)$$

and the conditional expectation of X given Y:

$$E\{X|Y=y\} = \sum_x x\, f_{X|Y}(x|y)$$

If this expression is treated as a function of the random variable Y, it then follows that:

$$E\{X\} = E\{E\{X|Y=y\}\} = \sum_y E\{X|Y=y\} \cdot f_Y(y)$$

$$= \sum_y \left\{ \sum_x x\, f_{X|Y}(x|y) \right\} f_Y(y)$$

$$= \sum_x x \left\{ \sum_y f_{X|Y}(x|y) \cdot f_Y(y) \right\} = \sum_x x\, f_X(x)$$

Example: (continued) First, work out the expectation of Y:

$$E\{Y\} = \sum_{y=0}^{\infty} y\, \frac{\lambda^y \exp\{-\lambda\}}{y!} = \lambda$$

By an exactly identical calculation, it follows from the fact that X is distributed according to a Poisson density with parameter $\lambda\rho$ that:

$$E\{X\} = \lambda\rho$$

However, even if we were unable to work out $f_X(x)$, we could use:

$$E\{X|Y=y\} = \sum_{x=0}^{y} x \binom{y}{x} \rho^x (1-\rho)^{y-x}$$

$$= \sum_{x=1}^{y} y \binom{y-1}{x-1} \rho^x (1-\rho)^{y-x} = y\rho$$

We could then use the result derived above to eliminate the conditioning:

$$E\{X\} = E\{E\{X|Y=y\}\} = \sum_{y=0}^{\infty} y\rho \cdot \frac{\lambda^y \exp\{-\lambda\}}{y!} = \lambda\rho$$

This is of course the same result we found earlier, but it was found by means of a simpler calculation.

We next proceed to consider the variance. It is well known that:

$$V\{Y\} = E\{[Y - E\{Y\}]^2\} = E\{Y^2\} - E\{Y\}^2$$

By analogy, we define the conditional variance:

$$V\{X|Y=y\} = E\{[X - E\{X|Y=y\}]^2 | Y=y\}$$
$$= E\{X^2|Y=y\} - E\{X|Y=y\}^2$$

As before, consider $V\{X|Y=y\}$ as a function of the random variable Y. Call this random function $V\{X|Y\}$. Since it is a function of a random variable, it has an expectation, $E\{V\{X|Y\}\}$. Similarly, the function $E\{X|Y\}$ has a variance, $V\{E\{X|Y\}\}$. In general, $E\{V\{X|Y\}\} \neq V\{E\{X|Y\}\}$.

We now proceed to show that:

$$V\{X\} = V\{E\{X|Y\}\} + E\{V\{X|Y\}\}$$
$$= E\{E\{X|Y\} - E[E\{X|Y\}]\}^2 + E\{E[X-E\{X|Y\}]^2|Y\}$$
$$= E[E\{X|Y\}-E\{X\}]^2 + E\{E\{[X^2-2XE\{X|Y\}+E\{X|Y\}^2]|Y\}\}$$
$$= E[E\{X|Y\}^2 - 2E\{X\}E\{X|Y\} + E\{X\}^2]$$
$$\qquad\qquad +E[E\{X^2|Y\} - 2E\{X|Y\}^2 + E\{X|Y\}^2]$$
$$= E\{X^2\} - E\{X\}^2 = V\{X\}$$

Example: (continued) We first calculate the variance of Y:

$$V\{Y\} = E\{Y^2\} - E\{Y\}^2$$

$$\rightarrow \quad V\{Y\} = \sum_{y=0}^{\infty} y^2 \frac{\lambda^y \exp\{-\lambda\}}{y!} - \lambda^2 \quad \rightarrow \quad \lambda^2 + \lambda - \lambda^2 \quad = \lambda$$

Hence by means of an identical calculation, $V\{X\} = \lambda\rho$, since S is distributed according to a Poisson density with parameter $\lambda\rho$. Alternatively, we could first find:

$$V\{X|Y=y\} = \sum_{x=0}^{y} x^2 \binom{y}{x} \rho^x (1-\rho)^{y-x} - y^2\rho^2$$

$$\rightarrow \quad = y\rho(1-\rho)$$

And then find:

$$V\{X\} = E\{V\{X|Y=y\}\} + V\{E\{X|Y=y\}\}$$

$$= \rho(1-\rho)E\{Y\} + \rho^2 V\{Y\} = \lambda\rho$$

Problems

All problems refer to the following data:
$$S_0 = s_0 = 3, \quad I_0 = i_0 = 1, \quad q = 1/2, \quad N = 4$$

1. Use the deterministic model to estimate the fraction of the population which eventually contracts the disease, σ_∞.

2. Use the deterministic model to project the expected numbers of infectives and susceptibles for four time intervals.

3. Apply Method I to find the expected number of infectives and susceptibles for the duration of the epidemic.

4. Using the results of problem 3, calculate the probability that there will be R removals at the end of the epidemic.

5. Apply Method II to simulate the development of the epidemic. (Note: Although you would ordinarily consult a table of random numbers to do this simulation, to make answers uniform, use the following: First Random Mumber = 0.46
   Second Random Number = 0.65
   Third Random Number = 0.16
   Fourth Random Number = 0.80

6. Apply Method III to find the final size distribution of the epidemic. Compare these numbers with the ones you found in problem 4.

References

Most of the ideas in this section are due to Donald Ludwig; it is
therefore best to refer to his presentation:

Ludwig, D., <u>Stochastic Population Models</u>, Lecture notes in
Biomathematics, Volume 3, Springer-Verlag, New York, 1974.

The chain binomial model is discussed in section II-1. The
interested reader should consult the sections which discuss the
relationship of the chain binomial model to the general
stochastic epidemic. Note that this book has quite a few
typographical errors in the equations.

Chapter 5. Branching Process Model

In this chapter a stochastic model called a branching process is developed to describe a small outbreak of a contagious disease in a large susceptible population. We will imagine that one or several infectious individuals arrive in an otherwise disease-free area and start the outbreak. To avoid the situation in which the outbreak gets out of control and eventually involves all susceptibles in the population, we assume that conditions are sufficiently unfavorable that the outbreak never becomes very large.

A more realistic scenario is that a single infected individual imports a disease which at first spreads very rapidly. Once public health authorities realize that an epidemic has begun quarantine procedures are employed to make conditions unfavorable for further spread and the outbreak subsides. The branching process model best describes the outbreak after the introduction of public health measures but while there are still a number of unidentified infectives in the population.

The feature of the branching process model which distinguishes it from the other models studied thus far is the way the structure of the epidemic is visualized. Imagine that when the model begins there are K infectives in the population. Each of these individuals infects zero or one or two or ... additional individuals. If we perceive of the original infectives as forming the zeroth generation of the disease, then the people they infect are the first generation, and so forth for subsequent generations. The outbreak ends once all lines of the disease die out.

The figure below is a directed graph (digraph) representation for a typical small outbreak. The vertices in the digraph represent infected individuals and the edges represent paths of infection from the source to the recipient of the disease.

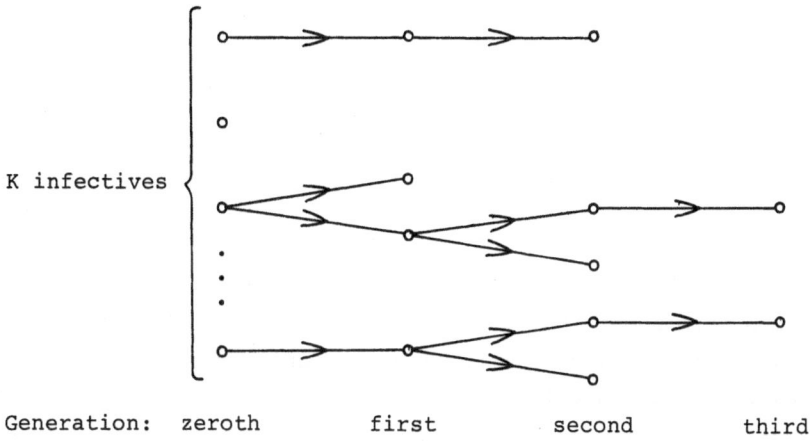

K infectives

Generation: zeroth   first   second   third

Disease Transmission Probability

The first problem to be considered is the disease transmission rate. The simplest reasonable assumption is that each individual with the disease spends a length of time t being infectious, where t is a continuous random variable which is exponentially distributed with parameter μ. Thus,

$$\text{Prob}\{\text{infectious for time t}\} = \mu e^{-\mu t}$$

During the time that the infective in question remains contagious, the disease is being spread to susceptible individuals. Assume that contacts sufficient to transmit the disease to susceptibles take place independently at random such that the average number of cases transmitted by one infective per unit time is λ.

It follows that for one infective the conditional probability of transmitting j cases, given that the contagious period lasts for t units of time, $P\{j|t\}$, is given by a time dependent Poisson density:

$$P\{j|t\} = \frac{(\lambda t)^j}{j!} \exp\{-\lambda t\}$$

n.b.   In the Appendix at the end of this chapter the relationship

between independent random occurrences, exponential inter-event
times and the Poisson density is carefully derived.

To eliminate the conditioning in $P\{j|t\}$, make use of the assumption
make earlier that the length of the infectious period is exponentially
distributed with parameter μ. Thus, the probability, p_j, that one
infective transmits j cases during his contagious period is:

$$p_j = \int_0^\infty \frac{(\lambda t)^j}{j!} \exp\{-\lambda t\} \cdot \mu \exp\{-\mu t\} \, dt$$

$$\rightarrow \quad = \left(\frac{\mu}{\lambda+\mu}\right)\left(\frac{\lambda}{\lambda+\mu}\right)^j$$

a result which follows by repeated integration by parts. Notice that
p_j is distributed according to a geometric density.

We will assume throughout the development of the model that the
number of cases of the disease transmitted by one particular victim
of the disease is independent of the number transmitted by any other
victim. Consider the ith infective, and let U_i be an integer-valued
random variable which counts the number of cases of the disease which
are transmitted by the ith infective. Since U_i is distributed
according to p_j, the expected number of new cases $E\{U_i\}$ is given by:

$$E\{U_i\} \equiv \theta = \sum_{j=0}^\infty j \, p_j = \frac{\lambda}{\mu}$$

Keeping the Disease Outbreak Small

It was stated in the introduction to this chapter that we imagine
conditions to be unfavorable for a major epidemic ; thus the disease
outbreak dies out quickly. Let us next determine what this means in
terms of our variables.

Consider one particular infective in the zeroth generation. Let d_m
be the probability that the portion of the outbreak developing from
the chosen infective has died out by the mth generation.

n.b. Clearly, for the whole outbreak to end, each of the K separate
      portions emanating from the K individual infectives in the
      zeroth generation must independently end.

Assume that the chosen infective in the zeroth generation (call him
the "father") infects j individuals (call them his "sons"). We could
view each son as the head of a line of the disease. If the fathers'

portion of the outbreak is to have ended by the $(m+1)^{st}$ generation, then the portion from each of the j sons must independently have ended after m additional generations of the disease have occurred. This occurs with probability equal to $[d_m]^j$. But since we do not know j, we must do an average over all choices of j, weighted by p_j, the probability that the father had j sons; hence

$$d_{m+1} = \sum_{j=0}^{\infty} p_j [d_m]^j = f(d_m)$$

We identify $f(d_m)$ as the probability generating function for the discrete density p_j.

The expression just found is a recurrence relation for the sequence $\{d_0, d_1, d_2, \ldots, d_m, d_{m+1}, \ldots\}$. We can make several observations:

1. Since d_m is the probability that a line of the epidemic has ended by the mth generation, it follows that

$$0 \leq d_0 \leq d_1 \leq d_2 \leq \cdots \leq d_m \leq d_{m+1} \leq \cdots \leq 1$$

2. Since the father of a line certainly has the disease, $d_0 = 0$; the probability that the father produces no sons (i.e. new infectives) is p_0, thus $d_1 = p_0$.

3. The sequence must approach a limit since it can never exceed unity in value, so

$$\lim_{m \to \infty} d_m \to d \leq 1$$

The third observation allows us to rewrite the recurrence relation as a non-recursive equation for d, the probability of ultimate extinction of one line of the disease:

$$d = f(d)$$

This result, which is true for any disease transmission probability, assumes a particularly simple form for the geometric density under study; equating d to the probability generating function for the geometric density determined earlier yields:

$$d = \frac{1}{1 + (1-d)\lambda/\mu}$$

Solving for d provides

$$d = \begin{cases} \mu/\lambda & \text{if } \lambda \geq \mu \\ 1 & \text{if } \lambda < \mu \end{cases}$$

n.b.   The two choices arise as the roots of a quadratic equation. The proper choice is always the smaller root which turns out to be the one satisfying $0 \leq d \leq 1$.

Finally, the probability that all of the branches of the epidemic started by the K individuals in the zeroth generation will independently die out is given by:

$$\text{Prob\{outbreak ends\}} = d^K = \begin{cases} \left(\frac{\mu}{\lambda}\right)^K & \text{if} \quad \lambda \geq \mu \\ 1 & \text{if} \quad \lambda < \mu \end{cases}$$

Thus, the condition for the outbreak to end with certainty is that $\lambda < \mu$. This is equivalent to the expected number of sons per father, θ, satisfying

$$\theta = \lambda/\mu < 1.$$

The Branching Process

The next step is to determine the number of individuals who ever contract the disease.

Recall that the infectives transmit the disease independently and that the number of cases transmitted by the ith infective, U_i, is distributed with the same geometric density as before, so

$$\text{Prob}\{U_i = j\} = p_j$$

and

$$E\{U_i\} = \theta$$

Next, define W_m to be an integer valued random variable which counts the total number of infectives in the mth disease generation who follow directly from one particular infective in the zeroth generation. Since these individuals each received the disease from one of the W_{m-1} infectives in the $(m-1)^{st}$ generation, it follows that

$$W_m = \sum_{i=1}^{W_{m-1}} U_i$$

The expected value of W_m follows easily from the conditional expectation given W_{m-1}; hence

$$E\{W_m\} = E[E\{W_m | W_{m-1}\}]$$
$$= E[E\{\sum_{i=1}^{W_{m-1}} U_i | W_{m-1}\}]$$

But the expected value of a sum equals the sum of the expected values, so

$$E\{W_m\} = E[\sum_{i=1}^{W_{m-1}} E\{U_i\} | W_{m-1}]$$

$$= E[\Theta W_{m-1}]$$

Since Θ is a constant, this may be rewritten as a simple difference equation

$$E\{W_m\} = \Theta E\{W_{m-1}\}$$

This is easily solved by using induction, and the fact that $E\{W_0\} = 1$ (since the model counts the number of infectives who develop from a single infective in the zeroth disease generation); thus

$$E\{W_m\} = \Theta^m \quad : m = 0,1,2,\ldots$$

We must next add up the expected number of infectives in all successive generations. The total number resulting for all K infectives in the zeroth generation, N, is just K times the number resulting from a single infective, thus:

$$N = K \sum_{m=0}^{\infty} \Theta^m = \frac{K}{1-\Theta} = \frac{\mu K}{\mu - \lambda}$$

since $\Theta = \lambda/\mu$.

n.b. We have succeeded in finding the expected number of individuals who ever contract the disease without ever finding the underlying probability density.

Although the quantity N is the one we ordinarily wish to know, it is instructive to work out the probability that exactly n_K people are involved in the disease outbreak.

Begin by defining q_n to be the probability that the line of the disease which develops from one particular infective in the zeroth disease generation contains exactly n infectives.

Conceptually what we will do is to draw all possible disease digraphs (starting from a single individual) which contain exactly n infectives and then add up the probability that each occurs. To do so we will need one more bit of notation. Let v_j be the number of individuals who infect exactly j others; using the terminology of graph theory, v_j is the number of vertices in the disease digraph with outgoing degree equal to j.

It is not difficult to see that for any connected disease digraph (starting from a single individual) which involves n infectives, the v_j must satisfy:

$$\sum_{j=0}^{n} v_j = n \qquad \text{and} \qquad \sum_{j=0}^{n} j v_j = n - 1$$

Next, let $\alpha(n; v_0, v_1, \ldots, v_n)$ be the number of disease digraphs involving n infectives, such that v_j infect exactly j others, with $j = 0, 1, 2, \ldots, n$. Notice that for compatible choices of the v_j, the quantity $\alpha(n; v_0, v_1, \ldots, v_n)$ accounts for all possible forms of the disease digraph.

Since the probability that a particular individual will infect j others is p_j, the probability that v_j individuals will independently each infect j others is p_j raised to the power v_j. Consequently, the probability that a line of the epidemic developing from a single individual contains exactly n infectives, q_n, is the sum over all disease digraph configurations times the probability that the configuration occurs; thus

$$q_n = \sum \alpha(n; v_0, v_1, \ldots, v_n) \, p_0^{v_0} \, p_1^{v_1} \cdots p_n^{v_n}$$

where the sum is carried out over all sets v_j; $j = 0, 1, \ldots, n$ for which

$$\sum_{j=0}^{n} v_j = n \qquad \text{and} \qquad \sum_{j=0}^{n} j v_j = n - 1$$

n.b. We could actually perform this sum, though to do so we would need to know $\alpha(n; v_0, v_1, \ldots, v_n)$. Although finding it provides an interesting exercise in combinatorics, we will not do so here as a more general method is available.

We will proceed now to define the probability generating function $g(y)$ for the q_n:

$$g(y) = \sum_{n=0}^{\infty} q_n \, y^n$$

and then relate $g(y)$ to $f(x)$, the probability generating function for the geometric density p_j. The relationship is found by means of a clever change of variables.

Let

$$p^*_j \equiv p_j x^j / f(x) \qquad\qquad : j = 0, 1, 2, \ldots$$

where we imagine x to be a real constant whose value will be chosen shortly. Also, define q^*_n in terms of p^*_j by analogy with the way q_n was defined in terms of p_j. That is,

$$q^*_n = \sum \alpha(n; \nu_0, \nu_1, \ldots, \nu_n) \; p^{*\nu_0}_0 \; p^{*\nu_1}_1 \cdots p^{*\nu_n}_n$$

$$= q_n x^{n-1} / [f(x)]^n$$

Defining the probability generating function, $g^*(w)$, for the q^*_n leads to:

$$g^*(w) = \sum_{n=0}^{\infty} q^*_n w^n \quad = \quad \frac{1}{x} \sum_{n=0}^{\infty} q_n [wx/f(x)]^n$$

$$= \frac{1}{x} g [wx/f(x)]$$

and setting $y = wx/f(x)$ provides

$$g(y) = x \, g^*[y \, f(x)/x]$$

This is the crucial expression.

First, realize that since g* is a probability generating function, $g^*(1) = 1$. We therefore select $x = \bar{x}$ such that the argument of g* is unity. This provides two expressions:

$$\bar{x} = y \, f(\bar{x})$$

and $$\bar{x} = g(y)$$

n.b. The first equation can be solved for x as a function of y; but the second equation says that this function is in fact the probability generating function for the q_n.

Using the probability generating function for the geometric density, $f(x)$, in the first equation results in a quadratic equation whose solution is

$$\bar{x} = \frac{\lambda+\mu}{2\lambda} \left[1 - \sqrt{1 - \frac{4\lambda\mu \, y}{(\lambda+\mu)^2}} \right] = g(y)$$

Expanding the expression under the square root using the binomial series, and comparing the result with the series definition of g(y) yields

$$q_n = - \frac{\lambda+\mu}{2\lambda} \binom{1/2}{n} [-4\lambda\mu/(\lambda+\mu)^2]^n \quad : n = 1, 2, \ldots$$

Recall that q_n is the probability that one infective in the zeroth disease generation creates a line containing n infectives. Since

there are K independent infectives in the zeroth generation, the
probability generating function for the entire disease outbreak, Q(y),
is simply

$$Q(y) = [g(y)]^K$$

Although we can formally substitute the expression for g(y) from
above, it is not possible to write a simple series expression for
Q(y). We can however verify the consistency of the result by using
Q(y) to calculate the expected number of individuals involved in the
disease outbreak; recall that this quantity, which was called N, was
found earlier:

$$N = \frac{dQ}{dy}\bigg|_{y=1} = K\frac{dg}{dy}\bigg|_{y=1} = \frac{\mu K}{\mu - \lambda}$$

This completes the analysis of the branching process model for a small
epidemic.

Appendix

This appendix will illustrate the relationship between independent
random events, exponential inter-event times, and the time-dependent
Poisson density.

Let X(t) be an integer valued random variable which serves as a
counter; thus each time an "event" occurs X(t) is incremented by one.
Assume that at $t = 0$, the counter is set to zero, so $X(0) = 0$.

The central ssumption is that events occur independently at random.
By this we mean the following: Imagine that time is subdivided into
small intervals of length Δt. The probability that one event occurs
in a particular interval of length Δt is $\gamma \Delta t$. Because we may make Δt
as small as we wish, we may ignore the possibility of more than one
event in an interval. Thus, the probability that no event occurs in
an interval of length Δt is $(1 - \gamma \Delta t)$. In addition, all non-
overlapping time intervals are independent of one another.

n.b. Intuitively this means that the occurrence of an event at one
     particular instant of time neither increases nor decreases the
     likelihood of occurrence of another event at any other time.

We will now calculate the probability density for the random variable
X(t); thus let

$$\text{Prob}\{X(t) = n\} = p_n(t) \qquad : n = 0, 1, 2, \ldots$$

Suppose that we wish to find $p_n(t + \Delta t)$ for $n = 1, 2, \ldots$. There are two mutually exclusive situations at time t which permit this:

1. At time t, $X(t) = n - 1$ with probability $p_{n-1}(t)$ and during the next time interval of length Δt an event occurs with probability $\gamma \Delta t$.

2. At time t, $X(t) = n$ with probability $p_n(t)$ and during the next interval of length Δt, no event occurs with probability $(1 - \gamma \Delta t)$.

Since these two alternatives are mutually exclusive and exhaustive, they can be written in the form

$$p_n(t + \Delta t) = p_{n-1}(t) \gamma \Delta t + p_n(t)(1 - \gamma \Delta t)$$

Rearranging, and taking the limit as $\Delta t \to 0$ leads to

$$\frac{dp_n(t)}{dt} = \gamma [p_{n-1}(t) - p_n(t)] \qquad : n = 1, 2, \ldots$$

If $n = 0$, an argument like the one above leads to the equation

$$\frac{dp_0(t)}{dt} = -\gamma p_0(t)$$

Since $X(0) = 0$, it follows that $p_0(0) = 1$ and $p_n(0) = 0$ for $n = 1, 2, \ldots$ These expressions serve as initial conditions for the set of equations just derived.

Although a variety of procedures are available to solve this system of equations, the simplest is a successive method. Separating and integrating the differential equation for $p_0(t)$ along with its initial condition provides

$$p_0(t) = \exp\{-\gamma t\}$$

Next, set $n = 1$ in the differential-difference equation and substitute $p_0(t)$ from above to get

$$\frac{dp_1(t)}{dt} + \gamma p_1(t) = \gamma \exp\{-\gamma t\}$$

But notice that if one multiplies both sides by the integrating factor $\exp\{\gamma t\}$, this can be rewritten

$$d[p_1(t) \exp\{-\gamma t\}] = \gamma \, dt$$

which integrates along with the initital condition $p_1(0) = 0$ to give

$$p_1(t) = \gamma t \exp\{-\gamma t\}$$

Repeating the same procedure which worked for $n = 1$ inductively leads to the general result

$$P_n(t) = \frac{(\gamma t)^n \exp\{-\gamma t\}}{n!} \qquad : n = 0, 1, 2, \ldots$$

This is the well known time dependent Poisson density function which describes the probability that by time t, exactly n random events have occurred.

Notice next that $p_0(\tau) = \exp\{-\gamma\tau\}$ is the probability that the first event has not occurred by time $t = \tau$, or in other words, that the first event takes place after time τ. Thus the distribution function for the first event occurring before time τ is

$$F(\tau) = 1 - \exp\{-\gamma\tau\}$$

and the derivative

$$f(\tau) = \frac{dF(\tau)}{d\tau} = \gamma \exp\{-\gamma\tau\}$$

is the density function for the first event occurring at time τ.

Perhaps the most interesting aspect of this result is that it is independent of where the zero point of time is located. Thus, if $\tau = 0$ is chosen to correspond with one event, then $f(\tau)$ is the probability density for the time of occurrence of the next event.

In summary, when events occur independently at random, the probability density for the length of time between events is exponential and the probability density for the number of events by a given time is Poisson.

Problems:

1. Use repeated integration by parts to show that

$$\int_0^\infty \frac{(\lambda t)^j e^{-\lambda t}}{j!} \mu e^{-\mu t} \, dt = \left(\frac{\mu}{\lambda+\mu}\right)\left(\frac{\lambda}{\lambda+\mu}\right)^j \equiv p_j$$

2. Given the geometric density p_j in problem 1, find the associated probability generating function, $f(x)$, and use this to calculate the expected value of j.

3. Given that ν_k is the number of individuals in an epidemic who transmit k cases of the disease and that a line of an epidemic started by a single individual involves n people in all,

    a. Show that

$$\sum_{k=0}^n \nu_k = n$$

b. Show that

$$\sum_{k=0}^{n} k \nu_k = n - 1$$

4. Given the expression

$$\bar{x} = y f(\bar{x}) = g(y) = \sum_{n=0}^{\infty} q_n y^n$$

where $f(\bar{x})$ is the probability generating function derived in problem 2,

a. Solve for $g(y)$.

b. Expand $g(y)$ in a binomial series to find q_n.

5. Imagine that a small epidemic is introduced by a single disease importer. If the average number of cases transmitted by one infective, $\theta = 2/3$

a. Estimate the expected size of the outbreak.

b. Find the probability, q_n, that exactly n individuals are involved in the outbreak, for n = 0, 1, 2, 3.

References

It is possible to find a treatment of simple branching processes in most books on stochastic processes. Unfortunately, these are all too often rather opaque; one pleasant exception is noted below:

Kemeny, J.G. and J.L. Snell, Mathematical Models in the Social Sciences, M.I.T. Press, Cambridge, Massachusetts, 1972.

Chapter 7, which is entitled "Branching Processes," provides a lucid discussion of the solution method employed here. The combinatorial procedure for evaluating the probability that the branching process involves n individuals is carefully explained in Appendix E.

Chapter 6. Smallpox Vaccination Discontinuation

In this section we consider the application of stochastic epidemic
theory to a real problem. The question to be addressed is: when
should routine vaccination against a rare disease be discontinued?
This question will be discussed in terms of smallpox, though the ideas
can be extended to a variety of other diseases.

Some facts about smallpox

1. Smallpox is a terrible disease; 10% of those who contract it
    die, and those who survive are usually badly scarred.

2. Not a single case of smallpox has occurred in the United
    States since 1949. In fact, since the disease appears to
    have been eradicated from the earth, no more cases will occur.

3. In 1968, 14,168,000 people were vaccinated against smallpox
    in the United States at a cost of $150,000,000. There were
    572 cases of "complications" due to the vaccine and 9 deaths.

Although it is now obvious that the smallpox vaccination is pointless,
we would like to know at what level of disease risk versus vaccine
risk it becomes prudent to discontinue routine vaccination. We could
approach this from the economic viewpoint of minimizing total cost in
dollars, or the medical viewpoint of minimizing loss of life. Since
the role of preventive medicine has always been to prevent suffering,
we choose the latter.

Brief history of smallpox

It has been known since ancient times that smallpox creates its own
natural immunity. If one survives a case of the disease then one is
immune in the future. Early efforts at disease prevention consisted
of innoculating susceptible individuals with material drawn from a
pustule on the body of an active case, a technique called variolation.
(The latin name for smallpox is variola major.) At the beginning of
the eighteenth century, Edward Jenner started using a related virus,
the one which causes cowpox, to provide immunity to smallpox. This
technique, which persists to the present time with only minor
modification, is called vaccination. It is interesting to note that
the first incidence of mathematical modelling in the field of
epidemiology concerned the effectiveness of Jenner's technique. The
study was presented by the famous Swiss mathematician Daniel Bernoulli
in 1760 before the French Royal Academy of Sciences. In 1958, the
World Health Organization undertook a campaign to eradicate the
disease from the earth. The last naturally transmitted case appears
to have occurred on 26 October 1977 in Somalia.

The epidemiology of smallpox

Smallpox is a highly contagious disease which is transmitted only
among humans — there is no known animal reservoir. About 10% of all
cases prove fatal. The incubation period appears to be random in
length, but to average about 1 to 2 weeks. During this period, the
disease is asymptomatic but contagious. With modern means of travel,
this implies that the disease could innocently be carried to any point
on earth. Once smallpox is identified, at least in the developed part
of the world, it is easily contained by isolation and contact tracing.
Consequently, if an epidemic did get started in the United States, it
could be brought under control rather quickly. As an example, in 1970
a case of smallpox was imported to Meschede, West Germany. The small
epidemic which resulted included 17 cases with 4 deaths.

The mathematical model

The mathematical model will consist of three separate pieces which
will subsequently be linked together.

> 1. The Pre-epidemic Period: During this phase there are
>   no cases of the disease, and routine vaccination takes
>   place at a level sufficient to maintain a prescribed
>   degree of population immunity.

2. The Epidemic Initiation Period: During this period the
    disease is imported by an unsuspecting carrier, and
    spreads until the first case is identified and isolated.

3. The Epidemic Subsistence Period: During this phase, the
    disease continues to spread through natural
    infectiousness, but is brought under control through
    contact tracing and isolation of suspected infectives.
    The epidemic runs its course, never becoming very large.

We proceed now to look at the three stages of the epidemic in detail.

The Pre-epidemic Model

Consider a large population in which nobody has smallpox. Assume for
the sake of simplicity that the population is fixed in size with a
total of N individuals, and that the daily probability of disease
importation is a constant, $\alpha \ll 1$.

If the disease is imported on the rth day for the first time, then for
$r - 1$ days the population is disease-free. The probability that this
occurs is:

$$\text{Prob\{disease imported on } r^{th} \text{ day\}} \equiv P_r = (1 - \alpha)^{r-1}\alpha$$

It is easily verified that this is a proper probability density, and
that the expected waiting time to disease importation is thus:

$$E\{r\} = \sum_{r=0}^{\infty} r\, P_r = \frac{1}{\alpha}$$

n.b. Although α itself is hard to estimate, the expected waiting time
      between importations is easier to assess, and thus provides an
      estimate of $1/\alpha$.

Next, consider the vaccination program which is used to maintain the
level of susceptibility at a prestated goal. Let

$\quad$ V $\;=\;$ number of vaccinations per day

$\quad$ β $\;=\;$ probability of death due to vaccination

It then follows that the probability that m individuals will die due
to vaccination during a period of r days is Binomially distributed:

$$\text{Prob\{m}|r\} = \binom{rV}{m} \beta^m (1 - \beta)^{rV-m}$$

and the conditional expected number of deaths due to vaccination
during a period of r days is:

$$E\{m|r\} = \sum_{m=0}^{rV} m \cdot \text{Prob}\{m|r\} = \beta rV$$

But this quantity may be viewed as a function of the random variable r, and thus its unconditional expectation may be found:

$$E\{m\} = \sum_{r=0}^{\infty} E\{m|r\} \cdot P_r = \frac{\beta V}{\alpha}$$

But $V = V(s)$, where s is the fraction of the population which is susceptible. Note that since nobody has the disease, the remaining fraction, $1 - s$, of the population is immune. In order to keep the model fairly simple, make the following assumptions:

1. A fraction ℓ of the population survives for 1 more year.

2. Vaccine-induced immunity lasts for k years.

3. Since the population size is fixed at N, the number of births and immigrants equals the number of deaths and emigrants.

4. Survival and susceptibility are independent variables.

5. All newborns and immigrants are susceptible.

The easiest way to visualize the evolution of susceptibility is to make a table:

	Initially Susceptible	Initially Immune
Survive 1 year:	$Ns\ell$	$N(1-s)\ell$
Die or depart:	$Ns(1-\ell)$	$N(1-s)(1-\ell)$

To maintain a fixed level of susceptibility:

1. Immunize $(1 - s)$ of all newborns and immigrants.

2. Immunize $1/k$ of all initially immune individuals.

Since the number of births and immigrants equals the number of deaths and emigrants, the first of the above two groups requires $N(1-s)(1-\ell)$ vaccinations per year. The number of vaccinations required to maintain the immunity of the second group is $N(1-s)\ell/k$. Thus

$$V(s) = N(1 - s)[1 - \ell + \ell/k]/365 \text{ vaccinations/day}$$

And the expected number of vaccine-related deaths prior to disease importation which was found earlier becomes:

$$E\{m\} = \frac{\beta N (1 - s)}{\alpha} [1 - \ell + \ell/k]/365$$

The Epidemic Initiation Model

The epidemic begins when an individual with smallpox arrives from abroad to a disease-free area. The individual arrives unnoticed, so the epidemic initially grows out of control. Let

Y(t) = number of unidentified infectives at time t

Since the average time to discovery of the disease is rather short, at worst only a tiny fraction of the population will become infected before the disease is identified and countermeasures are taken. We therefore proceed to make the following assumptions:

1. The population at risk is effectively infinite in size.

2. The latent period (time from initial contact until contagiousness develops) is zero, and the incubation period (time from development of contagiousness until externally observable symptoms become apparent) is exponentially distributed.

n.b. It was shown in the Appendix to Chapter 5 that if any infective is as likely as any other to be the first to manifest externally observable symptoms, the duration of the incubation period for individuals is exponentially distributed.

These assumptions suggest that the initial phase of the epidemic be modelled by means of a stochastic Birth-Death process, where in the present context "birth" corresponds with a contact which leads to a new case of the disease and "death" corresponds with the identification and subsequent isolation of one case of the disease.

To specify the governing equation for a Birth-Death process, it is necessary to determine the probability of a new case ("birth") or a discovery ("death") during a short interval of time Δt.

1. The rate of production of new infectives occurs in proportion to the number of unidentified infectives, Y(t), the number of susceptibles, Ns = n, and a proportionality constant, λ, which depends upon social customs:

    $$\text{Prob}\{Y \to Y+1\} = \lambda n Y(t) \Delta t$$

2. Discovery of the disease occurs soon after one of the asymptomatic individuals manifests symptoms. Since each

of the $Y(t)$ unidentified infectives has the same chance
of being discovered, if the probability for each
individual of discovery per unit time is ω,

$$\text{Prob}\{Y \to Y-1\} = \omega Y(t) \Delta t$$

At this point we could easily derive the governing equation for the
stochastic Birth-Death process. However, its solution would tell us
the probability that $Y(t) = y$. This is not what we wish to know. What
we want to determine is the expected value of $Y(t)$ when the first
discovery takes place.

The desired result is simple to determine once it is recognized that
imbedded within the Birth-Death process is a simple Random Walk which
is in fact independent of explicit clock time.

n.b. A Random Walk is a type of Markov Chain in which there are just
   two transition probabilities. Here, one corresponds with adding
   another unidentified infective, the other corresponds with
   discovering the disease.

The transition probabilities are easily determined from the
transition probabilities for the Birth-Death process:

$$\text{Prob}\{\text{additional infective}\} = \frac{\lambda n Y(t) \Delta t}{\lambda n Y(t) \Delta t + \omega Y(t) \Delta t} = \frac{\lambda n}{\lambda n + \omega}$$

$$\text{Prob}\{\text{identification}\} = \frac{\omega Y(t) \Delta t}{\lambda n Y(t) \Delta t + \omega Y(t) \Delta t} = \frac{\omega}{\lambda n + \omega}$$

n.b. Since these two quantities are mutually exclusive and exhaustive,
   they sum to unity. In addition, they are independent of both
   time and number of unidentified infectives:

It is now a straightforward operation to find the probability P_y that
there are $y-1$ additional unidentified infectives beyond the initial
disease importer (and thus a total of y infectives) followed by the
identification of one of these infectives:

$$P_y = \left(\frac{\lambda n}{\lambda n + \omega}\right)^{y-1} \left(\frac{\omega}{\lambda n + \omega}\right)$$

Since this is just a geometric density, its expectation is readily
found to be:

$$E\{Y\} = \sum_{y=0}^{\infty} y \, P_y = \frac{\lambda n + \omega}{\omega}$$

At this point in the epidemic there are $y-1$ additional unidentified
infectives and one identified case. Contact tracing and isolation

change the nature of the epidemic process; while contagion remains
the same, removal occurs at a greatly accelerated pace since suspected
infectives are quarantined to halt the spread of the disease.

The Epidemic Subsidence Model

n.b. The mathematical model discussed in Chapter 5, a Small Stochastic
Epidemic, could be used directly for this phase of the epidemic.
For the sake of variety, a completely different model is used
instead. Both models give identical results.

In addition to the random variable, $Y(t)$, which counts the present
number of unidentified infectives at time t, we will need another
random variable which counts the (cumulative) number of cases of
smallpox beyond the initial importer of the disease. Let

$Z(t)$ = number of cases of smallpox beyond the initial case
at time t

n.b. Since it will be assumed that the epidemic is always brought
under control, $Y(t) \to 0$ as $t \to \infty$. In fact, once the first case of
the disease is identified, $Y(t)$ is a generally decreasing
function of time. On the other hand, $Z(t)$ only increases since
it counts total cases.

Knowing about the existence of the disease mobilizes a massive public
health campaign. This consists of contact tracing and quarantine.
While this does not affect the natural contagiousness of the disease,
it drastically increases the removal rate. Anyone suspected of
contact with an infected individual is isolated. This means that we
need to define a new removal rate, μ, which plays the same role here
as ω played in the epidemic initiation model, and $\mu \gg \omega$.

The transition probabilities defined in the previous section can now
be generalized as follows:

$$\text{Prob}\{Y \to Y+1;\ Z \to Z+1\} \ = \ \lambda n Y(t) \Delta t$$

$$\text{Prob}\{Y \to Y-1;\ Z \to Z\} \ = \ \mu Y(t) \Delta t$$

n.b. When a new case develops, both Y and Z increase by one; when a
new case is removed, Y decreases by one but Z remains the same.

We next derive the Differential-Difference Equation for the Multi-
Birth-Death process. Notice that the variable we are really
interested in is $Z(t)$, since deaths due to the epidemic will depend
upon total cases. However, the disease dynamics depend upon the
current number of unidentified infectives, hence we must also keep

track of $Y(t)$.

To proceed, define:

$$p_{y,z}(t) = \text{Prob}\{Y(t) = y; \ Z(t) = z\}$$

and consider the situations which lead to $p_{y,z}(t+\Delta t)$. There are three mutually exclusive cases:

1. Epidemic is at $Y(t) = Y - 1$, $Z(t) = z - 1$, and a new case develops with probability $\lambda n(y-1)\Delta t$.

2. Epidemic is at $Y(t) = y + 1$, $Z(t) = z$, and an unidentified infective is removed with probability $\mu n(y+1)\Delta t$.

3. Epidemic is at $Y(t) = y$, $Z(t) = z$, and neither a new case nor a removal occurs with probability $1 - (\lambda n + \mu)y\Delta t$.

Introducing the respective probabilities for the three exclusive cases leads to the relation:

$$p_{y,z}(t+\Delta t) = \lambda n(y-1)\Delta t \cdot p_{y-1,z-1}(t) + \mu(y+1)\Delta t \cdot p_{y+1,z}(t)$$

$$+[1 - (\lambda n + \mu)y\Delta t] \cdot p_{y,z}(t)$$

Rearranging, and letting $\Delta t \to 0$ leads to the Differential-Difference Equation:

$$p'_{y,z} = \lambda n(y - 1)p_{y-1,z-1} - (\lambda n + \mu)\, y\, p_{y,z} + \mu(y+1)\, p_{y+1,z}$$

where prime denotes differentiation with respect to time.

We could solve this equation, but only with considerable difficulty; fortunately, all that is required is a knowlege of the expected total number of people who have contracted smallpox after the epidemic ends. In order to find this quantity, begin by defining the expectations:

$$E\{Y(t)\} = \sum_{y=0}^{\infty} \sum_{z=0}^{\infty} y\, p_{y,z} \qquad \& \qquad E\{Z(t)\} = \sum_{y=0}^{\infty} \sum_{z=0}^{\infty} z\, p_{y,z}$$

Thus

$$E'\{Y(t)\} = \sum_{y=0}^{\infty} \sum_{z=0}^{\infty} y\, p'_{y,z} \qquad \& \qquad E'\{Z(t)\} = \sum_{y=0}^{\infty} \sum_{z=0}^{\infty} z\, p'_{y,z}$$

Substitute the Differential-Difference Equation into these two expressions, and work out the sums formally. The first leads to the Differential Equation:

$$E'\{Y(t)\} = (\lambda n - \mu)E\{Y(t)\}$$

which can be separated and integrated to yield:

$$E\{Y(t)\} = E\{Y(0+)\}\exp\{(\lambda n - \mu)t\}$$

where $E\{Y(0+)\}$ is the number of unidentified infectives in the population just after the first infective is identified.

n.b. Since $E\{Y(t)\} \to 0$ as $t \to \infty$, this implies that $\mu > \lambda n$.

The second Differential Equation is:

$$E'\{Z(t)\} = \lambda n E\{Y(t)\}$$

Substituting $E\{Y(t)\}$ from above, and integrating leads to:

$$E\{Z(t)\} = K + E\{Y(0+)\} \frac{\lambda n}{\lambda n - \mu} \exp\{(\lambda n - \mu)t\}$$

where K is a constant of integration.

To evaluate the constant of integration, make use of the fact that $E\{Z(0+)\} = E\{Y(0+)\}$.

Finally, to find the number of individuals beyond the disease importer who contract smallpox, find the limiting value of $E\{Z(t)\}$ as $t \to \infty$. Since $\mu > \lambda n$, it is readily concluded that:

$$\lim_{t \to \infty} E\{Z(t)\} = K = \frac{\mu}{\mu - \lambda n} E\{Y(0+)\}$$

Optimal Vaccination Policy

The more one vaccinates the more people die from the vaccine, but the less severe the epidemic when it occurs. In order to estimate the optimal vaccination rate, we consider one 'cycle' consisting of the long waiting period before the disease importer arrives during which all deaths are due to the vaccine, and then the short epidemic during which all deaths are due to the disease.

Combining the results of all three models, we find that the expected number of total deaths, D(s), during one cycle is:

$$D(s) = \frac{\beta N}{\alpha} \cdot \frac{1 - \ell + \ell/k}{365} (1 - s) + \nu[1 + \frac{\mu \lambda Ns}{(\mu - \lambda Ns)\omega}]$$

where ν is the fraction of smallpox victims who die from the disease. Note that the first term is D(s) represents the deaths due to the vaccine. Clearly, if $s = 1$, nobody is vaccinated, and hence no deaths occur. The second term is D(s) represents deaths due to the disease, and accounts for the disease importer and all subsequent cases. Clearly, if $s = 0$, everybody is vaccinated and only the disease importer may die.

To establish the vaccination rate which minimizes total deaths, set

$$\frac{dD(s)}{ds} = 0 \quad \rightarrow \quad s = s*$$

On physical grounds, $0 \leq s* \leq 1$. It then follows that

$$s* = \begin{cases} 0 \text{ if } 365\alpha\lambda\nu > \omega\beta[1 - \ell + \ell/k] \\ \min\left[\frac{\mu}{\lambda N}[1 - \{\frac{365\alpha\lambda\nu}{\omega\beta(1-\ell+\ell/k)}\}^{\frac{1}{2}}], 1\right] \text{ :otherwise} \end{cases}$$

Implications of Model

In order to assess the implications of the model, it is necessary to estimate the parameters. We do so using rough arguments as follows:

α: Since $1/\alpha$ = expected waiting time for disease importation, based upon experiences of the developed nations of the world, it seems reasonable to expect an outbreak once every three years, or about once every 1000 days. Thus, let $\alpha = 1/1000 = 10^{-3}$.

β: Since about one person per million vaccinated dies from the vaccine, let $\beta = 10^{-6}$.

ℓ: In the developed nations of the world, one finds that about 99% of the population survives for one more year, hence $\ell = .99$

k: Standard revaccination periods range from 3 to 5 years. We will choose the average, and let $k = 4$.

N: The population of the United States is slightly in excess of 215 million. For simplicity, let $N = 2 \times 10^8$

ω: Since $1/\omega$ = expected waiting time until the first case of the disease is discovered, and since this is thought to be about a week, let $\omega = .2$

μ: Since $1/\mu$ = expected waiting time until new cases are removed, under the best conditions this is probably ten times faster than discovering the first case, hence let $\mu = 2.0$

ν: Since on average one person in ten who contracts smallpox dies from the disease, let $\nu = 0.1$

λ: The disease transmission rate will be treated as a parameter. If everyone is susceptible, each infective would transmit λN cases on average per day. In U.S. $\lambda N \simeq 1$.

Shown below is a plot of s* versus λN for the data given above.

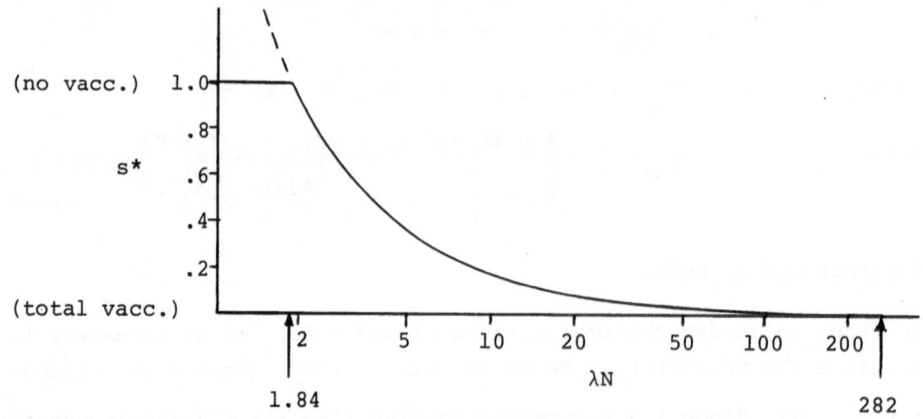

Notice that the implication is that for as long as this data has been reasonable (which is probably the past 20 years) the United States vaccination program has killed more people than would have been expected to die from the disease.

Note that the model does not pertain to medical personnel, or to individuals who would be travelling in smallpox endemic areas. It only suggests that we waited too long to stop vaccinating the average American. This observation was of course supported by the fact that no cases of the disease have been imported in thirty years, making disease immunity immaterial.

Problems

1. Assuming that the probability that the disease is first imported on the rth day is given by $p_r = (1 - \alpha)^{r-1}\alpha$, show that the expected waiting time to the first importation is given by $E\{r\} = 1/\alpha$.

2. If the probability of m vaccine-caused deaths given that vaccination is continued for r days is

$$\text{Prob}\{m|r\} = \binom{rV}{m} \beta^m (1 - \beta)^{rV-m}$$

   show that the conditional expected number of deaths is $E\{m|r\} = \beta r V$.

3. Using the expression from problem 1 for p_r in the result found in problem 2 for $E\{m|r\}$, show that $E\{m\} = (\beta V)/\alpha$.

4. It is claimed in the Epidemic Initiation Model that the length of the incubation period for each infected individual is

exponentially distributed with parameter ω. Show that this implies that the expected duration of the incubation period is then $1/\omega$.

5.   Starting from the transition probabilities:

$$\text{Prob}\{Y \to Y+1\} = \lambda n Y(t) \Delta t$$

$$\text{Prob}\{Y \to Y-1\} = \omega Y(t) \Delta t$$

and the definition $p_Y(t) = \text{Prob}\{Y(t) = Y\}$, derive a Differential-Difference Equation for the Birth-Death process.

6.   Given the difinitions

$$E\{Y\} = \sum_{y=0}^{\infty} \sum_{z=0}^{\infty} y\, p_{y,z}$$

$$E\{Z\} = \sum_{y=0}^{\infty} \sum_{z=0}^{\infty} z\, p_{y,z}$$

and the Differential-Difference Equation

$$\frac{d}{dt} p_{y,z} = \lambda n (y-1) p_{y-1,z-1} - (\lambda n+\mu) y\, p_{y,z} + \mu (y+1) p_{y+1,z}$$

differentiate the definitions and substitute the Differential-Difference Equation to derive

$$\frac{d}{dt} E\{Y\} = (\lambda n - \mu) E\{Y\}$$

$$\frac{d}{dt} E\{Z\} = \lambda n E\{Y\}$$

7.   Given that

$$D(s) = \frac{\beta N}{\alpha} \frac{1 - \ell + \ell/k}{365} (1 - s) + \gamma [1 + \frac{\mu \lambda N s}{\omega (\mu - \lambda N s)}]$$

Find the critical value $s = s*$ where $D(s)$ reaches a minimum.

References

The model analyzed in this section was originally proposed in the technical literature by Becker, and subsequently represented by Bailey. The specific references are:

Bailey, N,T,J., The Mathematical Theory of Infectious Diseases, Hafner Press, New York, 1975.

The models and a considerable amount of background material can be found in chapter 20 of this very comprehensive textbook.

Becker, N., "Vaccination Programmes for Rare Infectious Diseases," Biometrika, Volume 59, Number 2, pp. 443-453, 1972.

This is a very readable account of the model by its original
proposer. In several places, the mathematical treatment is
somewhat more advanced than in the present presentation.

Brown, G.C. (ed.) "Is Routine Vaccination Necessary in the United
States?" A Symposium, <u>American Journal of Epidemiology</u>, Volume
93, Number 4, pp. 222-252, 1971.

This symposium contains seven separate papers by medical doctors
and public health workers. It presents several different
viewpoints and a great deal of interesting information about
smallpox, including a detailed account of the small epidemic
in Mechede, West Germany in 1970.

Langer, W.L., "Immunization Against Smallpox Before Jenner,"
<u>Scientific American</u>, Volume 234, Number 1, pp. 112-117, 1976.

This is an extremely readable account of the circumstances which
led to the adoption of variolation in Europe and the United
States, as well as the early stages of Jenner's discovery.

Chapter 7: Schistosomiasis Eradication

Schistosomiasis is one of the most widespread of all human diseases.
Roughly 200 million individuals, especially in the warmer climates of
the world, have the disease. The epidemiology of schistosomiasis is
rather complicated, and is best visualized as consisting of two
stages. In the first, flatworms (circariae) enter through the skin
of a human who swims or bathes in infected water. Male and female
worms mate within the human, and lay eggs in the blood vessls which
line the bladder and intestine. These eggs produce an immune reaction
which causes swelling of the spleen and liver, as well as chronic
heart disease. A portion of the eggs are excreted and find their way
back into the water supply, where they hatch into a larva called a
miricidium.

In the second stage of the disease, the miricidium invade the bodies
of snails. The infected snails then release a large number of
circariae, which are produced within their bodies by asexual means.
The circariae swim freely, and eventually penetrate the skin of a
human to repeat the cycle.

Because the snails play a vital role in the epidemiology of
schistosomiasis, and because nobody really cares much about snails,
the disease can be combated by poisoning the snails. Our interest is
drawn to this problem in part by the observation that snail
eradication projects tend to be far less effective in reducing human
schistosomiasis than would be naively expected. Modest eradication
programs have virtually no effect on the extent of infection in humans.

We will construct a model to explain this curious observation.
Although is is quite possible to look at models for various stages of
the disease, our model will focus upon the sexual reproductive phase
within the human host, as this appears to be the critical link.

The Basic Model

As much as possible, we will build a deterministic model so that it is
tractable. We will assume the following:

1. Essentially all humans who swim and bathe in infected
   water harbor circariae, and the number of these worms per
   human depends upon the concentration in the water supply.

2. The number of humans and the number of snails are
   effectively constant. The total number of humans will
   never enter the equations explicitly; the number of
   snails will appear as a parameter. Snail eradication
   programs will change this number, but not in a time-
   dependent manner within the model.

3. Since the phase of the reproductive cycle which occurs
   within the snails is asexual, we will assume that all
   infected snails are equally infected, and hence all
   release circariae at the same rate.

Let time, t, be a continuous variable, and let:

$n(t)$ = number of infected snails at time t

N = total number of snails

δ = death rate for infected snails

m = mean number of worms infecting each human

$\beta(m)$ = number of uninfected snails which become infected per
unit time per uninfected snail.

It follows directly from these definitions that the rate of change in
the number of infected snails is the rate at which uninfected snails
become infected less the rate at which infected snails die.
In symbols,

$$\frac{dn}{dt} = \beta(m)(N - n) - \delta n$$

We next recognize that the snail infection rate, $\beta(m)$, is really just
a measure of the rate at which humans excrete flatworm eggs, which is
in turn proportional to the mean number of sexually reproducing paired

flatworms within human hosts. Thus, let:

> P(m) = mean number of sexually reproducing paired flatworms
>   within a human
>
> B = a proportionality constant, defined such that:
>
> $\beta(m) = B\ P(m)$

The final equation describes the rate of change in the mean number of
worms per human host. Let:

> r = death rate for worms within humans
>
> A = a proportionality constant which measures the rate
>   at which circariae are produced by infected snails,
>   and then penetrate the skin of humans.

Reasoning as before, the rate of change in the mean number of worms
per human is:

$$\frac{dm}{dt} = An - rm$$

Before continuing, let us stop briefly to consider the parameters in
the model. The death rate for infected snails, δ, would be increased
by a snail eradication program. The proportionality constant B
relates egg output from human hosts to snail infections; hence a
comprehensive sanitation program would cause B to decrease. The worm
death rate within human hosts, r, would be increased by a program
which concentrates on human medical treatment. There is a very
effective drug called hycanthone which appears to kill virtually all
worms within humans; unfortunately, it also seems to cause cancer.
The proportionality constant A relates circariae production by
infected snails to human worm concentration; thus a campaign to kill
snails decreases A. We assume that we do not have a direct control
over either m or n, and that N is a constant.

The Flatworm Mating Model

We must next come to grips with the analytic form of P(m), the mean
number of sexually reproducing paired flatworms per human host, as a
function of m, the mean number of flatworms per human. The idea here
is that if m is very small, worms will not manage to find mates as
successfully as if m is large. This part of the model clearly must be
probabilistic in nature.

We make the following assumptions:

1. If the circulatory system of a human is visualized as being subdivided in many small regions, the number of worms within any region is independent of the number in any non-overlapping region.

2. If the size of a region is small (say ten times the size of a worm) then the probability of exactly one worm in a region is proportional to the size of the region, with the constant of proportionality called λ.

3. If the size of a region is small, then the probability of more than one worm being in that region is negligible in comparison with the probability of one worm.

n.b. By comparing these assumptions for a region of space (within a human) with those made in the Appendix to Chapter 5 for a period of time, it is apparent that the probability density which results from the assumptions is a Poisson density of the form

$$P_j = \frac{\lambda^j}{j!} \exp\{-\lambda\} \quad : \quad j = 0, 1, 2, \ldots$$

with expectation equal to λ.

Recall that we have defined m to be the expected number of worms per human host. If we assume that the expected number of males and of females is equal, each equals m/2. If we assume further that the numbers of males and of females are independent random variables, each with a Poisson density, then:

$$\text{Prob}\{p \text{ males}\} = \frac{(m/2)^p}{p!} \exp\{-m/2\}$$

$$\text{Prob}\{q \text{ females}\} = \frac{(m/2)^q}{q!} \exp\{-m/2\}$$

and thus,

$$\text{Prob}\{p \text{ males \& } q \text{ females}\} = \frac{(m/2)^{p+q}}{p! \, q!} \exp\{-m\}$$

Determination of P(m)

The species of flatworms which are involved with schistosomiasis have and unusual lifestyle. For most of the adult phase, the broad, flat male worm is wrapped around the tubelike female. Consequently, the number of sexually reproducing pairs of worms which will be formed is determined by whichever sex is in smaller supply. In other words, the number of paired parasites depends upon the function, min{p,q}, and takes the form:

$$P(m) = \sum_{p=0}^{\infty} \sum_{q=0}^{\infty} 2 \min\{p,q\} \exp\{-m\} \frac{(m/2)^{p+q}}{p! \; q!}$$

Although it is possible to evaluate this summation in terms on the
Modified Bessel Functions, we will instead look just at the limiting
behavior for small and large m. Clearly, if m << 1, then m >> m^2 >>
m^3 >> ···, so exp{-m} = 1 - m + ··· ≃ 1. Thus, the only term in the
double summation which is not either zero or of higher degree than
two in m is the one corresponding with p = q = 1; hence

$$P(m) \simeq m^2/2 \quad : \quad m \text{ small}$$

According to the Central Limit Theorem, as m gets large, the Poisson
density approaches a Normal density with mean and variance both equal
to m/2. Thus, replacing the name p for the number of male worms
with x, a continuous variable defined over the whole interval
from -∞ to +∞,

$$\text{Prob}\{x \text{ males}\} \simeq \frac{1}{\sqrt{m\pi}} \exp\{-(x - \frac{m}{2})^2 / m\}$$

and a similar expression for the probability of y female worms. It
then follows that:

$$\text{Prob}\{x \text{ males \& y females}\} \simeq \frac{1}{m\pi} \exp\{-[(x - \frac{m}{2})^2 + (y - \frac{m}{2})^2]/m\}$$

Next, using this approximate form to redefine the quantity P(m), we
arrive at

$$P(m) \simeq \frac{2}{m\pi} \int_{-\infty}^{+\infty} \int_{-\infty}^{+\infty} \min\{x,y\} \exp\{-[(x - \frac{m}{2})^2 + (y - \frac{m}{2})^2] / m\} \, dx \, dy$$

This is clearly an integral over the whole (x,y) plane of an integrand
which is symmetric in the variables x and y. We may use this
observation to replace min{x,y} by y itself if we double the integrand
and change the limits so that y ≤ x. This amounts to doing the
integral only over the half of the (x,y) plane below the line x=y.
The integral becomes

$$P(m) \simeq \frac{4}{m\pi} \int_{0}^{\infty} \int_{0}^{x} y \exp\{-[(x - \frac{m}{2})^2 + (y - \frac{m}{2})^2] / m\} \, dy \, dx$$

It is most convenient to shift the origin of coordinates to the point
(m/2, m/2) and then to transform to polar coordinates.

Defining

$$r^2 = (x - m/2)^2 + (y - m/2)^2$$

$$\theta = \tan^{-1}\left[\frac{y - m/2}{x - m/2}\right]$$

leads to

$$P(m) \simeq \frac{4}{m\pi} \int_{-3\pi/4}^{\pi/4} \int_0^\infty (\frac{m}{2} + r \sin\theta) \exp\{-r^2/m\}\, r\, dr\, d\theta$$

$$= m[1 - \sqrt{2/\pi m}] \quad \text{as} \quad m \to \infty$$

We are now in a position to assess the behavior of the model. Since we do not have a convenient analytic representation for $P(m)$, we will be forced to do so graphically.

Behavior of the Model

Begin by recalling the form of the basic model:

$$\frac{dm}{dt} = A n - r m$$

$$\frac{dn}{dt} = B P(m) \cdot (N - n) - \delta n$$

$$P(m) \sim \begin{cases} m^2/2 & \text{as } m \to 0 \\ m & \text{as } m \to \infty \end{cases}$$

Perform the graphical analysis by first locating the isoclines along which $dm/dt = 0$ and $dn/dt = 0$:

$$\frac{dm}{dt} = 0 \quad \to \quad n = \frac{r}{A} m \qquad \text{: a straight line through origin}$$

$$\frac{dn}{dt} = 0 \quad \to \quad n = \frac{N B P(m)}{B P(m) + \delta} \quad \sim \begin{cases} N B m^2/2\delta & \text{as } m \to 0 \\ N & \text{as } m \to \infty \end{cases}$$

It is also clear from the differential equations that:

$$\frac{dm}{dt} \gtrless 0 \quad \text{for } n \gtrless \frac{r}{A} m \quad \text{and} \quad \frac{dn}{dt} \gtrless 0 \quad \text{for } n \gtrless \frac{N B P(m)}{B P(m) + \delta}$$

This information is plotted in the figure below for choices of the parameters which lead to endemic schistosomiasis (as will be clear shortly.) The lines labeled $dm/dt = 0$ and $dn/dt = 0$ are the isoclines. The short arrows across the isoclines show the direction of the tangent to a solution trajectory as it crosses the isocline. The longer, curved lines represent typical solution trajectories.

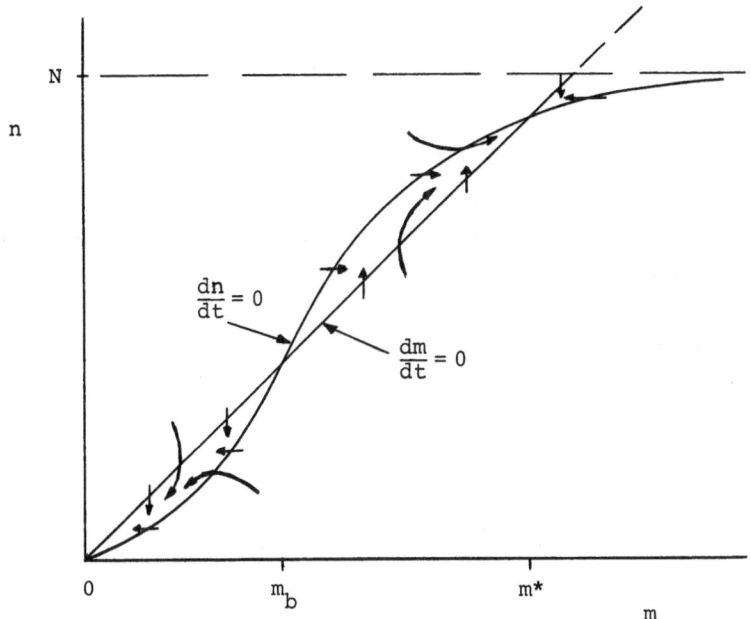

The two isoclines intersect at three equilibrium points, $m = 0$, $m = m_b$, and $m = m^*$. It is clear from the direction of the arrows that $m = 0$ and $m = m^*$ are stable points, and $m = m_b$ is an unstable point. Notice further that once the trajectory enters either of the long, narrow regions between the isoclines, it must remain within that region and eventually reach either $m = 0$ or $m = m^*$.

Interpretation of Results

The unstable equilibrium point, $m = m_b$, represents the "break-point." If m, the mean number of flatworms per individual in the population, can be made small enough so that the trajectory enters the long, narrow region between the isoclines and near to the origin, the solution will naturally approach the equilibrium at $m = 0$. However, if the solution is near to $m = m^*$, even substantial reductions in m will naturally return to $m = m^*$, the situation with the disease at its endemic level.

But recall that we do not control m directly; rather, we are able by public health measures to adjust the parameters (A, B, r and δ) which determine the location of the isoclines.

A major snail eradication program will have two effects: it will cause

A to decrease and δ to increase. These changes, respectively, cause the straight isocline to become steeper and the curved isocline to shift downward near to the origin. The results of a moderate snail eradication program are illustrated in the figure on the left. Notice that the effect of the shift in the isoclines is to increase the value of m_b and to decrease the value of m*. The results of a massive snail eradication program are shown in the figure on the right. Note that m_b and m* have coalesced, and then disappeared; the only equilibrium point which remains is at m = 0. The result is that schistosomiasis dies out spontaneously.

n.b.   We have been rather cavalier in our treatment of the constant N, the total number of snails. Obviously, a massive program to eradicate snails will change the value of N. It is not hard to show that N can be scaled so that its value is effectively unity without affecting the essential nature of the results. We are therefore justified in treating it as a constant here.

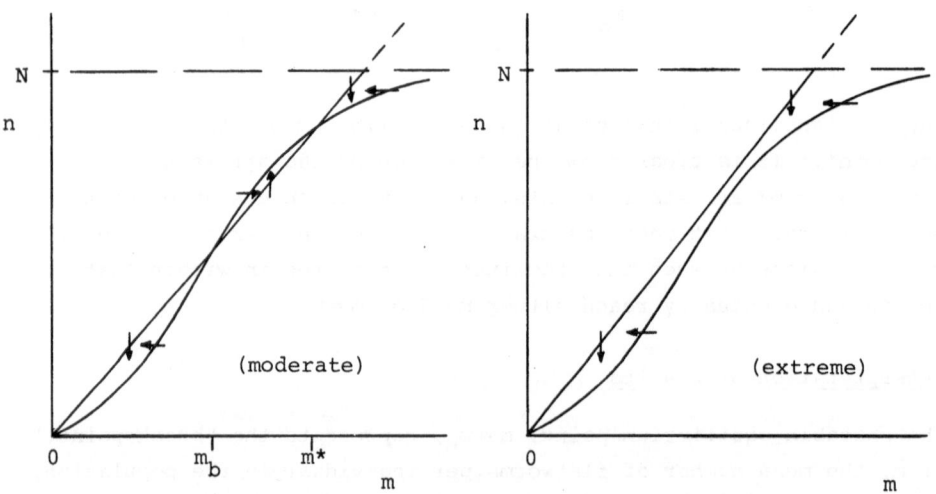

Our simple mathematical model has very successfully illustrated why it is that an insufficient snail eradication program has almost no effect on endemic schistosomiasis, while a sufficient program will lead to spontaneous disappearance of the disease. Clearly, if we wish to determine numerical values of the parameters necessary to cause the isoclines not to intersect, a more detailed model is required.

Problems

1.   Given: $p_j = \exp\{-m\}\, m^j / j!$

Show that:

$$\sum_{j=0}^{\infty} P_j = 1$$

2. Show by evaluating the integral that:

$$\frac{4}{m\pi} \int_{-3\pi/4}^{\pi/4} \int_{0}^{\infty} \left(\frac{m}{2} + r \sin \theta\right) \exp\{-r^2/m\} r \, dr \, d\theta = m[1 - \sqrt{2/\pi m}]$$

3. It was stated that once either of the long, narrow regions between the isoclines is entered by the solution trajectory, it cannot be left again. Carefully explain why this is true.

4. Given that the Modified Bessel Functions are defined by

$$I_\ell (m) = \sum_{j=0}^{\infty} \frac{(m/2)^{2j+\ell}}{j! \, (j+\ell)!} \quad : \ell \geq 0$$

Rewrite the earlier definition for the joint Poisson density in the form:

$$\text{Prob}\{p \text{ males \& } q \text{ females}\} = \exp\{-m\} \cdot a_{pq}$$

where

$$a_{pq} \equiv \frac{(m/2)^{p+q}}{p! \, q!}$$

and use this to show that

$$\sum_{\ell=-\infty}^{+\infty} I_\ell (m) = \exp\{m\}$$

Hint: Visualize a_{pq} as an infinite matrix, and consider sums down diagonals which run from upper left to lower right.

5. Show that

$$W_\ell (m) \equiv \sum_{j=0}^{\infty} \frac{j \, (m/2)^{2j+\ell}}{j! \, (j+\ell)!} = \frac{m}{2} I_{\ell+1} (m)$$

and then use this result along with the results of problem 4 to show that the number of sexually reproducing flatworms is:

$$P(m) = m \left[1 - \exp\{-m\}[I_0 (m) + I_1 (m)]\right]$$

6. It is well known that for large m, the Modified Bessel Functions may be approximated by the asymptotic expansion:

$$I_\ell (m) \sim \frac{\exp\{m\}}{\sqrt{2\pi m}} \left[1 - \frac{4\ell^2 - 1}{8m} + \cdots \right] \quad : \text{ as } \quad m \to \infty$$

Use this expression along with the definition of P(m) in problem
5 to show that

$$P(m) \sim m[1 - \sqrt{2/\pi m}] \quad : \quad \text{as } m \to \infty$$

References

The mathematical model discussed in this chapter originally appeared
in the literature of tropical medicine, though with somewhat less
mathematical elegance. The model was reformulated in an educational
form by Ludwig and Haytock. Additional models for schistosomiasis
can be found in a paper by Joel Cohen.

Cohen, J.E., "Mathematical Models of Schistosomiasis," Annual Review
of Ecological Systems, Volume 8, pp. 209 - 233, 1977.

Although the present model is not discussed in this paper, it
contains an excellent description of the epidemiology of the
disease, further models, and a large bibliography.

Ludwig, D and B.D. Haytock, "MacDonald's Work on Helminth Infections,"
Case Studies in Applied Mathematics, Mathematical Association
of America, Chapter 8, pp. 313 - 334, 1976.

This volume consists of a collection of interesting mathematical
models written for undergraduate students. The one by Ludwig
and Haycock contains a more extensive version of the present
model. Note that the paper by MacDonald, which forms the basis
of the model, is reprinted in its entirety in this volume.

MacDonald, G., "The Dynamics of Helminth Infections, with Special
Reference to Schistosomiasis," Transactions of the Royal Society
of Tropical Medicine and Hygiene, Volume 59, Number 5, 1965.

This paper is rather heavy reading, in part because it was
written for the tropical medicine community. The mathematical
formulation is considerably less well designed than in the
Ludwig-Haycock version.

Chapter 8. Gonorrhea

In this chapter we investigate a mathematical model for the spread of
gonorrhea, a highly contagious venereal disease. Over the past 25
years the incidence of the disease in the United States has risen
sharply, presumably due to changing sexual attitudes. Certain
contagious diseases such as hepatitis, mumps, rubella, syphilis, etc.,
must be reported by physicians to public health authorities. In
recent years reported cases of gonorrhea outnumber the total of all
other reportable diseases. It is estimated that each year 2,500,000
people in the United States contract gonorrhea. The goal of our model
will be to help us decide whether the recent rise in gonorrhea
incidence is the start of an epidemic or just a change in the endemic
level.

Epidemiology of Gonorrhea

Gonorrhea is spread by sexual contact and affects both males and
females. Within a few days after infection, males develop an itching
or burning sensation while urinating and an easily noticed discharge;
females often experience no symptoms. For both sexes sterility,
blindness, cardiac dysfunction, and eventually death may result if the
disease is not treated. Fortunately, gonorrhea responds well to
antibiotics, though no natural immunity is created by the disease, nor
is artificial immunity available.

The disease is unusual from an epidemiological viewpoint. With the
exception of a small number of cases transmitted between homosexuals,

the disease is passed back and forth between males and females by heterosexual contact.

n.b.   This is similar to the "host-vector" mechanism for the spread of schistosomiasis or malaria, except that now each sex serves as "vector" for the other.

It is somewhat difficult to decide on the actual number of individuals who are at risk of contracting gonorrhea. Clearly, celibate people and people who have contact only with non-infectives ("faithfully married couples," ...) will not contract the disease.   We will therefore consider in our model only heterosexual individuals who might contact gonorrhea.

The Mathematical Model

Assume that there are N_1 males and N_2 females at risk of, or infected with, gonorrhea, and assume that these numbers are constants.

n.b.   Changing sexual mores as well as natural population growth would cause these to vary slowly. Thus our model represents a "snapshot" of the situation at some particualr period in time.

Let

$I_1(t)$ = number of male infectives at time t

$I_2(t)$ = number of female infectives at time t

and since all individuals under consideration are either susceptible or infective,

$N_1 - I_1(t)$ = number of male susceptibles at time t

$N_2 - I_2(t)$ = number of female susceptibles at time t

Restating the epidemiology in the form of mathematical assumptions suggests:

1. Infectives are cured at a rate γ_1 which is proportional to I_1 for males, and at a rate γ_2 which is proportional to I_2 for females. Since males develop symptoms, $\gamma_1 \gg \gamma_2$.

2. New male infectives are created at a rate β_1 which is proportional to the product of the number of susceptible males, $N_1 - I_1$, and the number of infectious females, I_2. Similarly, new female infectives occur at a rate β_2 which is proportional to $N_2 - I_2$ and I_1.

Following the sort of argument proposed in Chapter 1 leads to the pair of coupled ordinary differential equations:

$$\frac{d}{dt} I_1(t) = -\gamma_1 I_1(t) + \beta_1 [N_1 - I_1(t)] I_2(t)$$

$$\frac{d}{dt} I_2(t) = -\gamma_2 I_2(t) + \beta_2 [N_2 - I_2(t)] I_1(t)$$

As is all too often the case, since these equations are non-linear we must resort to approximate methods.

Possible Solutions

Before attempting to analyze the gonorrhea model we review the types of solutions which might occur.

Since there are only two dependent variables, I_1 and I_2, it is convenient to visualize the solution as a curve or trajectory in the (I_1, I_2) plane, called the phase plane.

n.b. Explicit time dependence of the solution does not appear in the phase plane.

There are three possible types of trajectories:

1. The solution can grow without bound as time increases.

2. The solution can approach a fixed limit cycle around an equilibrium point.

3. The solution can approach a fixed equilibrium point.

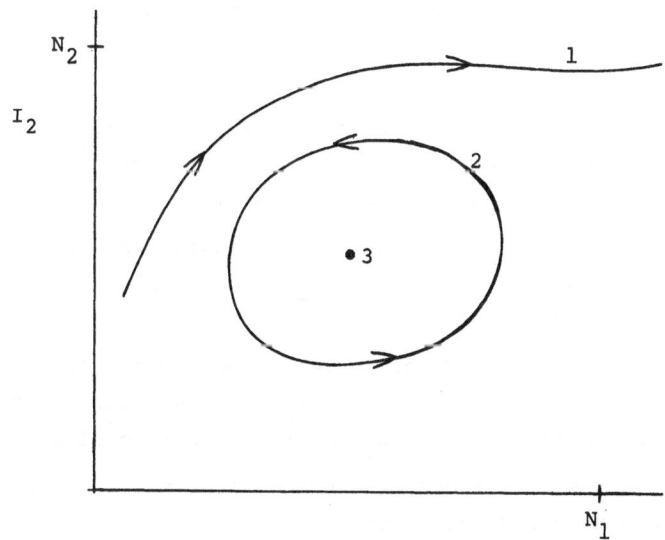

These three situations are illustrated above for a two dependent
variable system such as the one in the gonorrhea model: The arrows
indicate the direction of motion along the solution trajectory as time
passes, and the numbers refer to the three cases described above.

We begin by showing that the first case is not a possible solution for
our gonorrhea model. We do so by showing that the solution trajectory
must remain within the rectangle $\{0 \leq I_1 \leq N_1; \; 0 \leq I_2 \leq N_2\}$ in phase space if
it starts within this rectangle.

n.b.   Staying within the rectangle simply means that the number of
       infectives is somewhere between none and all of those individuals
       considered in the model to be at risk of infection.

Thus, assume that the model starts at time $t = t_0$, with $0 < I_1(t_0) < N_1$
and $0 < I_2(t_0) < N_2$.

We first show that if $I_1(t_0) > 0$ and $I_2(t_0) > 0$, then $I_1(t) > 0$ and
$I_2(t) > 0$ for all $t \geq t_0$. To do so, assume this is not true and let
$t* > t_0$ be the <u>first</u> time that I_1 or I_2 is zero. Say $I_1(t*) = 0$.
But from the first of the governing equations

$$\frac{d \, I_1}{dt} \bigg|_{t=t*} = \beta_1 N_1 I_2(t*) > 0$$

But this implies that just prior to $t = t*$, $I_1(t*-) < 0$ (and increases
to zero). But this is a contradiction. Since $I_1(t_0) > 0$, for $I_1(t*-)$
to be negative I_1 must have been zero at some time in the interval
$t_0 \leq t \leq t*$. But we assumed that $t*$ was the first time that I_1 was zero.
This shows that $I_1(t) > 0$ for all $t > t_0$. The same contradiction using
the second governing equation occurs for I_2.

n.b.   The above arguments do not apply when both $I_1 = 0$ and $I_2 = 0$.
       This of course corresponds with the situation where the disease
       is absent, and is a possible solution.

It is straightforward to modify the contradiction argument just
employed to show that if $I_1(t_0) < N_1$, and $I_2(t_0) < N_2$, then $I_1(t) < N_1$
and $I_2(t) < N_2$ for all $t > t_0$.

Thus we now know that our model yields realistic values for I_1 and I_2
so long as $0 < I_1(t_0) < N_1$ and $0 < I_2(t_0) < N_2$, though solutions like
the one labeled #1 in the figure above are not possible.

We next show that limit cycle solutions like the one labeled #2 in the
figure above also are not possible.

n.b.   The time trajectory corresponding with a closed orbit (limit

cycle) in phase space is a periodic oscillation. If the period
of the oscillation is T,

$$I_1(t) = I_1(t+T)$$
$$I_2(t) = I_2(t+T)$$

Recall that the governing equations can be written in the form

$$\frac{dI_1}{dt} = F_1(I_1,I_2)$$

$$\frac{dI_2}{dt} = F_2(I_1,I_2)$$

Assume that a periodic solution exists which can be represented in
phase space by a closed orbit C. Call the region which includes C
and its interior R. This is illustrated below:

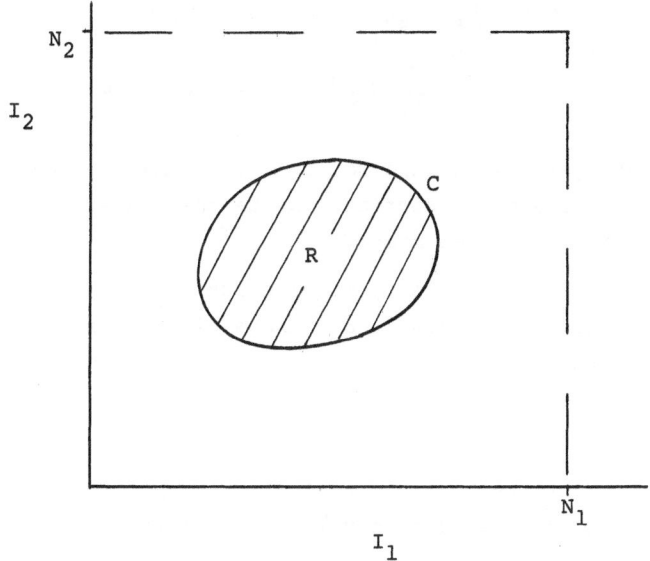

Lemma 1: Since C is a solution to the governing equations, along C

$$\frac{dI_1}{dt} = F_1(I_1,I_2) \qquad \text{and} \qquad \frac{dI_2}{dt} = F_2(I_1,I_2)$$

Thus

$$\oint_C [F_2\,dI_1 - F_1\,dI_2] = \int_0^T [F_2\frac{dI_1}{dt} - F_1\frac{dI_2}{dt}]\,dt$$

$$= \int_0^T [F_2F_1 - F_1F_2]\,dt = 0$$

where T is the period of C.

Lemma 2: From the expressions for F_1 and F_2 it follows easily that

$$\frac{\partial F_1}{\partial I_1} + \frac{\partial F_2}{\partial I_2} = -[\gamma_1 + \beta_1 I_2 + \gamma_2 + \beta_2 I_1] < 0$$

since all the quantities between the square brackets are positive.

Consequently

$$\iint\limits_R [\frac{\partial F_1}{\partial I_1} + \frac{\partial F_2}{\partial I_2}] \, dI_1 \, dI_2 < 0$$

It is now simple to show that no limit cycle C can exist. To do so use Green's Theorem in the plane to replace the double integral in Lemma 2 by a line integral around C:

$$0 > \iint\limits_R [\frac{\partial F_1}{\partial I_1} + \frac{\partial F_2}{\partial I_2}] \, dI_1 \, dI_2 =$$

$$\oint\limits_C [F_2 \, dI_1 - F_1 \, dI_2] = 0$$

where the final equality to zero follows from Lemma 1. But the expression above is a contradiction; hence there are no limit cycle solutions C to the gonorrhea model.

Having eliminated all possible types of solutions except fixed equilibrium points, we can now locate these with confidence that they represent the solution.

Stability Analysis

We will employ stability analysis to locate the possible equilibrium points and then to decide which equilibrium points are stable.

n.b. Physical systems which exhibit fixed point solutions will naturally tend to those equilibrium points which are stable. Thus, if there is only one stable point it represents the solution. If there is more than one stable point, then further analysis is required to decide which one attracts the solution.

Equilibrium:

The equilibrium points occur where

$$\frac{dI_1}{dt} = 0 \quad \text{and} \quad \frac{dI_2}{dt} = 0, \text{ simultaneously.}$$

From the governing equations we find the two expressions:

$$F_1(I_1, I_2) = 0 \rightarrow I_2 = \frac{\gamma_1 I_1}{\beta_1(N_1 - I_1)} \equiv f(I_1)$$

$$F_2(I_1, I_2) = 0 \rightarrow I_2 = \frac{\beta_2 N_2 I_1}{\gamma_2 + \beta_2 I_1} \equiv g(I_1)$$

which we solve simultaneously by setting $f(I_1) = g(I_1)$. Following a
bit of algebra we find that there are two possible equilibrium points:

$$\begin{bmatrix} I_1 = \bar{I}_1 = 0 \\ \\ I_2 = \bar{I}_2 = 0 \end{bmatrix} \quad \text{and} \quad \begin{bmatrix} I_1 = \bar{\bar{I}}_1 = \dfrac{\beta_1 \beta_2 N_1 N_2 - \gamma_1 \gamma_2}{\gamma_1 \beta_2 + \beta_1 \beta_2 N_2} \\ \\ I_2 = \bar{\bar{I}}_2 = \dfrac{\beta_1 \beta_2 N_1 N_2 - \gamma_1 \gamma_2}{\gamma_2 \beta_1 + \beta_1 \beta_2 N_1} \end{bmatrix}$$

Since we know that the solution must always remain in the rectangle
$\{ 0 \le I_1 \le N_1 \; ; \; 0 \le I_2 \le N_2 \}$, and since all parameters in the
expressions for $\bar{\bar{I}}_1$ and $\bar{\bar{I}}_2$ are positive, it follows that

1. If $\beta_1 \beta_2 N_1 N_2 \le \gamma_1 \gamma_2$, then the only allowable equilibrium
   point is at $(\bar{I}_1 = 0, \bar{I}_2 = 0)$.

2. If $\beta_1 \beta_2 N_1 N_2 > \gamma_1 \gamma_2$, then both equilibrium points are
   possible, so long as $\bar{\bar{I}}_1 \le N_1$ and $\bar{\bar{I}}_2 \le N_2$.

Stability:

We must next decide whether the solution will move to $(\bar{I}_1, \bar{I}_2)$ or to
$(\bar{\bar{I}}_1, \bar{\bar{I}}_2)$ when both are possible. To do so we will linearize the
governing equations around the equilibrium at $(0,0)$ as this is the
easiest way to proceed analytically. This amounts simply to deleting
the quadratic terms in the governing equations:

$$\left. \begin{array}{l} \dfrac{dI_1}{dt} = -\gamma_1 I_1 + \beta_1 N_1 I_2 \\ \\ \dfrac{dI_2}{dt} = \beta_2 N_2 I_1 - \gamma_1 I_2 \end{array} \right\} \quad : \; |I_1|, |I_2| \ll 1$$

Define the matrix quantities

$$\vec{X} = \begin{Bmatrix} I_1 \\ I_2 \end{Bmatrix}, \quad \underset{\sim}{M} = \begin{bmatrix} -\gamma_1 & \beta_1 N_1 \\ \beta_2 N_2 & -\gamma_2 \end{bmatrix}$$

and rewrite the linearized equations in compact form:

$$\dfrac{d\vec{X}}{dt} = \underset{\sim}{M} \vec{X}$$

Recall that linear, constant coefficient, ordinary differential
equations always have exponential solutions. Thus, substitute

$$\vec{X} = \{ {\textstyle A \atop \textstyle B} \} \exp\{\lambda t\} = \vec{K} \exp\{\lambda t\}$$

into the matrix equation. Upon rearranging this yields

$$[\underset{\sim}{M} - \lambda \underset{\sim}{I}] \vec{K} \exp\{\lambda t\} = 0 \quad : \underset{\sim}{I} = \begin{bmatrix} 1 & 0 \\ 0 & 1 \end{bmatrix}$$

Since $\exp\{\lambda t\} \neq 0$ in general, what remains is a set of homogeneous
algebraic equations. If these are to have a non-trivial solution, the
determinant of the coefficient matrix must be zero:

$$\det[\underset{\sim}{M} - \lambda \underset{\sim}{I}] = \lambda^2 = (\gamma_1 + \gamma_2) \lambda + \gamma_1 \gamma_2 - \beta_1 \beta_2 N_1 N_2 = 0$$

This is called the characteristic equation, and its roots determine
the stability. Employing the quadratic formula leads to

$$\lambda_{\frac{1}{2}} = \frac{1}{2}\{-(\gamma_1 + \gamma_2) \pm \sqrt{(\gamma_1 - \gamma_2)^2 + 4\beta_1 \beta_2 N_1 N_2}\}$$

It is apparent that both roots are always real, and

1. $\lambda_1 < 0, \quad \lambda_2 < 0 \quad$ if $\beta_1 \beta_2 N_1 N_2 < \gamma_1 \gamma_2$

2. $\lambda_1 > 0, \quad \lambda_2 < 0 \quad$ if $\beta_1 \beta_2 N_1 N_2 > \gamma_1 \gamma_2$

Since the solution is of the form

$$\begin{Bmatrix} I_1 \\ I_2 \end{Bmatrix} = \begin{Bmatrix} A_1 \\ B_1 \end{Bmatrix} \exp\{\lambda_1 t\} + \begin{Bmatrix} A_2 \\ B_2 \end{Bmatrix} \exp\{\lambda_2 t\}$$

where the A's and B's parameterize the initial small disturbance from
(0,0). It is clear from the nature of the roots λ_1 and λ_2 that (0,0)
is a stable equilibrium point if $\beta_1 \beta_2 N_1 N_2 < \gamma_1 \gamma_2$ and an unstable
equilibrium point if $\beta_1 \beta_2 N_1 N_2 < \gamma_1 \gamma_2$.

n.b. We could now analyze the local stability of the equilibrium at
$(\bar{\bar{I}}_1, \bar{\bar{I}}_2)$, but this is not really necessary. By a process of
elimination, it must be stable when (0,0) is unstable.

Conclusions

We are now prepared to understand why the incidence of gonorrhea has
risen recently. As noted in the introduction, changing sexual
attitudes have raised the values of N_1 and N_2, the number of males
and females at risk of or infected with the disease.·

Presumably, both now and in the past, the equilibrium point $(\bar{\bar{I}}_1, \bar{\bar{I}}_2)$

has been stable. As N_1 and N_2 increase, the location of this point moves further from the origin, and so the number of infectives increases.

However, using the words in their technical sense, gonorrhea is endemic at higher levels, but not undergoing an epidemic. For there to be an epidemic, it would be necessary for there to be a threshold which, if surpassed, would lead to an outbreak.

If we trust our model, then the only conclusion is that no such threshold exists. Once the values of N_1 and N_2 become constant, the number of infectives will stop growing.

Problems

1. Given the governing equations of the gonorrhea model:

$$\frac{dI_1}{dt} = -\gamma_1 I_1 + \beta_1 [N_1 - I_1] I_2$$

$$\frac{dI_2}{dt} = -\gamma_2 I_2 + \beta_2 [N_2 - I_2] I_1$$

   show that if $I_1(t_0) < N_1$ and $I_2(t_0) < N_2$ then $I_1(t) < N_1$ and $I_2(t) < N_2$ for all $t > t_0$.

2. Develop Green's Theorem in the plane for a simple, convex region R bounded by a closed curve C.

3. Employ the graphical method described in the chapter on schistosomiasis to analyze the stability of the gonorrhea model:

   a. For the case $\beta_1 \beta_2 N_1 N_2 > \gamma_1 \gamma_2$ which has two allowable equilibrium points.

   b. For the case $\beta_1 \beta_2 N_1 N_2 < \gamma_1 \gamma_2$ which has one allowable equilibrium point.

   Hint: Look at the relative slopes of the isoclines $I_2 = f(I_1)$ and $I_2 = g(I_1)$ at $(0,0)$ to help deduce how the isoclines intersect.

4. Homosexuals also contract gonorrhea. A model for the number of infectives $I(t)$ in a group of N interacting homosexuals is

$$\frac{dI}{dt} = -\gamma I + \beta [N - I] I$$

   where γ and β are the recovery and transmission rate constants.

   a. Locate all equilibrium points.

    b. When a non-zero endemic disease level I* is possible, find its stability using analytic techniques.

Hint: You should make the change of variables $I(t) = I* + x(t)$ and then linearize the resulting differential equation for $x(t)$.

5.   Imagine that the number of homosexuals at risk of, or infected with gonorrhea satisfies the differential equation

$$\frac{dN}{dt} = rN(1 - N/K) \quad : \quad r, \ K > 0$$

Using this along with the differential equation for the number of infectives from problem 4, deduce what happens as $t \to \infty$.

References

The model discussed in this chapter was learned from a similar educational treatment in a book by Martin Braun.

Braun, M., Differential Equations and Their Applications, Applied Mathematical Sciences Series, Vol. 15, Springer-Verlag, New York, 1975.

    This book contains a marvelously clear exposition of introductory differential equations along with many interesting models which are used as examples. The gonorrhea model is found in Chapter 4 Section 12.

Chapter 9. Sickle Cell Anemia

Sickle cell anemia is not an infectious disease, but rather a genetic
disorder. It is characterized by an abnormality in the hemoglobin
which causes the red blood cells to be deformed (sickle shaped
instead of flat). Victims' blood is not able to transport oxygen
properly and the vital organs are starved out; death occurs ordinarily
before reproductive maturity.

The disease is most common among individuals who live in the tropical
part of Africa. Since many American Blacks' ancestors came from that
part of the world, the disease sometimes affects these people.

Before we can understand sickle cell anemia, we must review some basic
genetics. Inherited traits are determined by proteins called genes.
Most genes occur in pairs, with one element of the pair coming from
each parent. The different possible forms of the genes are called
alleles, and certain traits — eye color for example — are determined
by a single gene with just one pair of alleles. Call the two alleles
A and a, and assume that the presence of the A allele causes the
individual to manifest the trait controlled by A. We therefore say
that A is dominant and a is recessive. Since individuals have a pair
of genes for the trait, three different genotypes can occur:

AA	Dominant Homozygote
Aa	Heterozygote
aa	Recessive Homozygote

n.b. The Aa and aA genotypes are identical — the order in which we write the alleles is irrelevant.

In the case of eye color, both the AA and Aa genotypes would have brown eyes; only the aa genotypes have blue eyes. The transmission of genes to offspring is determined by Mendel's Law of Inheritance. Before we look at the law, let us begin to formulate our model.

The Mathematical Model without Selection

Although humans reproduce in continuous time, it will be much easier to treat time as discrete and in units of one generation. We will imagine that we are looking at a population of fixed identity and determine the frequency (fraction) of genes (alleles) and genotypes in successive generations. Let

$$p_i = \text{fraction of A alleles in the } i^{th} \text{ generation}$$

$$q_i = \text{fraction of a alleles in the } i^{th} \text{ generation}$$

Consequently,

$$p_i + q_i = 1 \quad : \text{ all i}$$

Since we also wish to keep track of the genotype frequencies, we define a second set of variables which are not independent; let:

$$(D_i, H_i, R_i) = \text{fraction of (AA, Aa, aa) genotypes in the } i^{th} \text{ generation}$$

Once again,

$$D_i + H_i + R_i = 1 \quad : \text{ all i}$$

It is a simple matter to deduce the relationship between the gene frequencies and the genotype frequencies in any generation. Perhaps the easiest way to proceed is to imagine that there are N individuals in the population of the ith generation, and thus 2N genes in all. The total number of the A alleles will be $2ND_i$ from the dominant homozygotes and NH_i from the heterozygotes; hence

$$p_i = \frac{2ND_i + NH_i}{2N} = D_i + \frac{1}{2}H_i$$

Similarly,

$$q_i = \frac{2NR_i + NH_i}{2N} = R_i + \frac{1}{2}H_i$$

n.b. We will assume quite realistically that the gene frequencies (p_i, q_i) and genotype frequencies (D_i, H_i, R_i) are the same for males and females in the population, and further that mate selection takes place at random with respect to the trait in question.

Mendel's Law of Inheritance

Mendel's law says that the frequency of genotypes among the offspring
of parents of given genotypes obeys binomial proportions. For
example, imagine that a dominant homozygote and a heterozygote
reproduce. We denote this symbolically by

$$AA \times Aa \rightarrow \frac{(A+A)}{2} \frac{(A+a)}{2} = \frac{1}{2}AA + \frac{1}{2}Aa$$

and interpret this to mean that the offspring are half heterozygotes
and half dominant homozygotes.

Using this idea, we now extend our model to determine the genotype
frequencies in the $(i+1)^{st}$ generation given the genotype frequencies
in the ith generation. We do this most easily in tabular form:

Parent Genotype	Parent Frequency	Offspring Frequency AA	Aa	aa
AA × AA	D_i^2	D_i^2		
AA × Aa	$2D_i H_i$	$D_i H_i$	$D_i H_i$	
AA × aa	$2D_i R_i$		$2D_i R_i$	
Aa × Aa	H_i^2	$\frac{1}{4}H_i^2$	$\frac{1}{2}H_i^2$	$\frac{1}{4}H_i^2$
Aa × aa	$2H_i R_i$		$H_i R_i$	$H_i R_i$
aa × aa	R_i^2			R_i^2
Sums:	$(D_i+H_i+R_i)^2=1$	D_{i+1}	H_{i+1}	R_{i+1}

Reading from the final three columns of the table we have:

$$D_{i+1} = D_i^2 + D_i H_i + \frac{1}{4}H_i^2 = (D_i + \frac{1}{2}H_i)^2 = p_i^2$$

$$H_{i+1} = D_i H_i + 2D_i R_i + H_i R_i + \frac{1}{2}H_i^2 = 2(D_i+\frac{1}{2}H_i)(R_i+\frac{1}{2}H_i)$$
$$= 2p_i q_i$$

$$R_{i+1} = R_i^2 + R_i H_i + \frac{1}{4}H_i^2 = (R_i + \frac{1}{2}H_i)^2 = q_i^2$$

where the final equality results from the relationship between the
gene and the genotype frequencies. Using these for the $(i+1)^{st}$
generation yields:

$$p_{i+1} = D_{i+1} + \frac{1}{2}H_{i+1} = p_i^2 + p_i q_i = p_i$$

$$q_{i+1} = R_{i+1} + \frac{1}{2}H_{i+1} = q_i^2 + p_i q_i = q_i$$

$$\left.\right\} : \text{all } i$$

Hence we have learned that the gene frequencies remain unchanged from one generation to the next, starting with the initial group of individuals and carrying on through successive generations of their offspring. In other words, if the initial population has genotype frequencies $(D_0, H_0, R_0) \rightarrow (p_0, q_0)$, then:

$$(p_0, q_0) = (p_1, q_1) = (p_2, q_2) = \cdots$$

Further, since

$$D_{i+1} = p_0^2, \quad H_{i+1} = p_0 q_0, \quad R_{i+1} = q_0^2 \qquad : \text{all } i$$

$$(D_1, H_1, R_1) = (D_2, H_2, R_2) = (D_3, H_3, R_3) = \cdots$$

though in general these are not the same as (D_0, H_0, R_0).

In words, for any initial set of genotype frequencies, (D_0, H_0, R_0), which imply (p_0, q_0), if mating occurs at random, the gene frequencies never change and the genotype frequencies reach equilibrium after just one generation. This is called the Hardy-Weinberg Equilibrium.

The De Finetti Diagram

There is a convenient graphical representation of the genotype frequencies called the De Finetti Diagram. Draw an equilateral triangle with unit altitude, and label the vertices AA, Aa, and aa, as shown below. Then construct a line parallel to the side opposite the vertex labeled AA and a distance D away (toward the vertex). Do the same thing at a distance R away from the side opposite the vertex labeled aa. The intersection of these lines is H away from the side opposite the vertex Aa. Consequently, any point on or within the triangle represents a possible set of genotype frequencies for the population.

n.b. The gene frequency p is represented on the abscissa on a scale that runs from zero to one. The heterozygote frequency H is represented on the ordinate on a scale that also runs from zero to one. Since the De Finetti Diagram is superimposed on an equilateral triangle, it follows that unit length on the ordinate is shorter than unit length on the abscissa, and that D and R are measured using the ordinate scale.

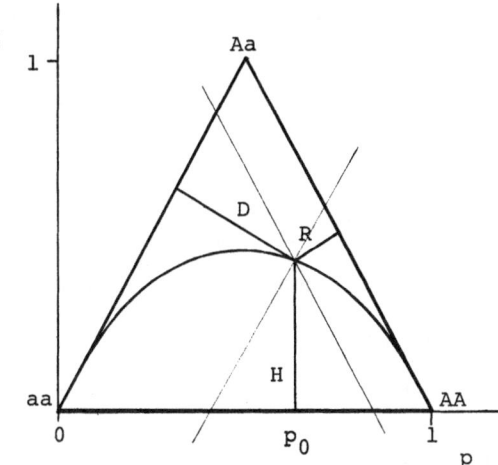

Since at the Hardy-Weinberg Equilibrium, $H_i = 2p_0q_0 = 2p_0(1-p_0)$, the parabola shown in the figure represents the locus of possible equilibrium points.

In addition, it is not hard to see that for any initial set of genotypes, (D_0, H_0, R_0), since the corresponding gene frequency, p_0, does not change, the point representing the genotype frequencies moves onto the parabola at a point vertically above or below the initial point after one generation of random mating.

The Mathematical Model with Selection

Although sickle cell anemia, like eye color, depends upon a single gene which has just two alleles (with the recessive homozygote causing the disease), our model does not suffice. This is because the recessive homozygote does not survive to reproduce; hence we must include in our model what geneticists call selection due to fitness. The fitness will be represented as the probability that an individual of the given genotype survives to reproduce, thus let

$$(W_{AA}, W_{Aa}, W_{aa}) = \text{the fitness of the genotype (AA, Aa, aa),}$$
$$\text{with } 0 \le W_{..} \le 1$$

If we start with gene frequencies (p_i, q_i), then immediately after the birth of the new generation, Mendel's Law tells us that

$$\bar{D}_{i+1} = p_i^2, \quad \bar{H}_{i+1} = 2p_iq_i, \quad \bar{R}_{i+1} = q_i^2$$

where
$$\bar{D}_{i+1} + \bar{H}_{i+1} + \bar{R}_{i+1} = 1$$

After selection due to the relative fitness of the genotypes occurs, these become

$$\bar{\bar{D}}_{i+1} = W_{AA}p_i^2, \quad \bar{\bar{H}}_{i+1} = 2W_{Aa}p_iq_i, \quad \bar{\bar{R}}_{i+1} = W_{aa}q_i^2$$

but now,
$$\bar{\bar{D}}_{i+1} + \bar{\bar{H}}_{i+1} + \bar{\bar{R}}_{i+1} \leq 1$$

with the equality only holding if $W_{AA} = W_{Aa} = W_{aa} = 1$.

Define the mean fitness in the ith generation, $\bar{W}_i$, as

$$\bar{W}_i = W_{AA}p_i^2 + 2W_{Aa}p_iq_i + W_{aa}q_i^2$$

and use this to renormalize the gene frequencies after selection:

$$D_{i+1} = \bar{\bar{D}}_{i+1}/\bar{W}_i = p_i^2 W_{AA}/\bar{W}_i$$

$$H_{i+1} = \bar{\bar{H}}_{i+1}/\bar{W}_i = 2p_iq_iW_{Aa}/\bar{W}i$$

$$R_{i+1} = \bar{\bar{R}}_{i+1}/\bar{W}_i = q_i^2 W_{aa}/\bar{W}_i$$

These are the genotype frequencies at the time of reproduction, and as a result of the renormalization,

$$D_{i+1} + H_{i+1} + R_{i+1} = 1$$

Further, since the relations:

$$p_i = D_i + \frac{1}{2}H_i \quad \text{and} \quad q_i = R_i + \frac{1}{2}H_i \quad : \text{ all } i$$

still hold, it follows that

$$p_{i+1} = (W_{AA}p_i^2 + W_{Aa}p_iq_i)/\bar{W}_i$$

$$q_{i+1} = (W_{aa}q_i^2 + W_{Aa}p_iq_i)/\bar{W}_i$$

It will turn out to be convenient to define still one more function of the fitness, the marginal mean frequencies for the individual alleles in the ith generation.

$$\bar{W}_{i,A} = W_{AA}p_i + W_{Aa}q_i$$

$$\bar{W}_{i,a} = W_{Aa}p_i + W_{aa}q_i$$

and thus:

$$p_{i+1} = p_i \bar{W}_{i,A} / \bar{W}_i \quad \text{and} \quad q_{i+1} = q_i \bar{W}_{i,a} / \bar{W}_i$$

n.b. If we substitute backwards, since $\bar{W}_i$, $\bar{W}_{i,A}$, and $\bar{W}_{i,a}$ all depend
   upon p_i and q_i, these are two coupled, nonlinear difference
   equations. For any given values of p_0 and q_0, as well as the
   fitnesses, W_{AA}, W_{Aa}, and W_{aa}, we could successively evaluate p_i
   and q_i.

Let us next ask where the equilibrium points are located. To do so,
set $p_{i+1} = p_i$ and $q_{i+1} = q_i$, simultaneously. The result is clearly

$$\bar{W}_{i,A} = \bar{W}_i = \bar{W}_{i,a}$$

From the definitions given above, it follows that

$$\bar{W}_i = p_i \bar{W}_{i,A} + q_i \bar{W}_{i,a}$$

and from this relation we can deduce two useful facts:

   1. At all times, either

$$\bar{W}_{i,A} \leq \bar{W}_i \leq \bar{W}_{i,a} \quad \text{or} \quad \bar{W}_{i,A} \geq \bar{W}_i \geq \bar{W}_{i,a}$$

   2. At equilibrium, which occurs when $\bar{W}_{i,A} = \bar{W}_{i,a}$, it will always
       happen that

$$\bar{W}_{i,A} = \bar{W}_i = \bar{W}_{i,a}$$

In order to find the location of this equilibrium in terms of the gene
frequencies, and also as an easy way to assess the stability, we
calculate the change in the frequency of the A allele between two
successive generations:

$$\Delta p_i \equiv p_{i+1} - p_i = p_i \bar{W}_{i,A} / \bar{W}_i - p_i$$

$$= p_i q_i (\bar{W}_{i,A} - \bar{W}_{i,a}) / \bar{W}_i$$

n.b. This expression provides us with several useful facts. It tells
   us that there will always be trivial equilibria at $p_0 = 0$ and at
   $q_0 = 0$. This is nothing more than the observation that if either
   allele is absent from the initial population, it will always
   remain absent. In addition, it tells us that as either p_i or q_i
   becomes close to zero, their rate of change also approaches zero.
   This means that selecting a gene out of existence is a very slow
   process.

There are three essentially different possible cases which depend upon
the relative magnitudes of the three genotype fitnesses. We first

list these and then sketch out the mathematical verification.

Case 1: $W_{AA} \geq W_{Aa} \geq W_{aa}$ (Purification)

It is not hard to show that in this case, $\bar{W}_{i,A} \geq \bar{W}_{i,a}$

→ $\Delta p_i \geq 0$: all $p_i \geq 0$.

This means that the fraction of the A allele keeps increasing in successive generations until the a allele is finally driven out entirely.

n.b. From the genetic point of view, this is an extremely profound result, as it provides a genetic basis for evolution. If some condition renders the marginal mean fitness of one allele smaller than the other, that form of the gene will slowly be driven to extinction.

Case 2: $W_{AA} < W_{Aa} > W_{aa}$ (Heterosis)

If we set $\bar{W}_{i,A} = \bar{W}_{i,a}$, which causes $\Delta p_i = 0$,

→ $p_i = p^* = \dfrac{\bar{W}_{aa} - \bar{W}_{Aa}}{\bar{W}_{AA} - 2\bar{W}_{Aa} + \bar{W}_{aa}}$, where $0 \leq p^* \leq 1$

n.b. This means that in addition to the trivial equilibria at $p_i = 0$ and $p_i = 1$, there is also an equilibrium at $p_i = p^*$

From the signs on the inequalities, it is not hard to deduce that:

$$p_i < p^* \quad \rightarrow \quad \Delta p_i > 0$$

and $\qquad p_i > p^* \quad \rightarrow \quad \Delta p_i < 0$

n.b. This means that the equilibrium at $p_i = p^*$ is stable.

Case 3: $W_{AA} > W_{Aa} < W_{aa}$ (Incompatibility)

This case is just case 2 with the signs reversed. Once again, there is an intermediate equilibrium at $p_i = p^*$, but this time it is unstable. If $p_0 < p^*$, the A allele is driven out, while if $p_0 > p^*$, the a allele is driven out.

Stability Analysis

Let us look a bit more carefully at the stability of the genetic equilibria for the three cases of Purification, Heterosis, and Incompatibility. To do so, first recall that:

$$\Delta p_i = p_i q_i (\bar{W}_{i,A} - \bar{W}_{i,a}) / \bar{W}_i$$

where $\qquad \overline{W}_i = p_i^2 W_{AA} + 2p_i q_i W_{Aa} + q_i^2 W_{aa}$

It is not difficult to show that the expression for Δp_i can be written in the form

$$\Delta p_i = \frac{p_i q_i}{2\overline{W}_i} \frac{d\overline{W}_i}{dp_i}$$

Equilibrium:

$$\Delta p_i = 0 \;\rightarrow\; \begin{cases} p_i = 0 \;\rightarrow\; q_i = 1 \\[2mm] q_i = 0 \;\rightarrow\; p_i = 1 \\[2mm] \dfrac{d\overline{W}_i}{dp_i} = 0 \;\rightarrow\; (p_i, q_i) = (p^*, q^*) \end{cases}$$

n.b. The first two equilibria occur for all three cases; the third one only occurs for cases 2 and 3 (Heterosis and Incompatibility). Clearly, this point corresponds with either a maximum or a minimum of the function $\overline{W}_i$. Since this function is quadratic in p_i, there can be at most one maximum or minimum.

Stability: To assess the stability of the equilibrium at (p^*, q^*), consider the quantity

$$\left.\frac{d \,\Delta p_i}{dp_i}\right|_{p^*} = \left.\frac{p_i q_i}{2\overline{W}_i} \frac{d^2 \overline{W}_i}{dp_i^2}\right|_{p^*}$$

It is not hard to show that this quantity is negative for the case of Heterosis and positive for the case of Incompatibility.

Graphical Analysis:

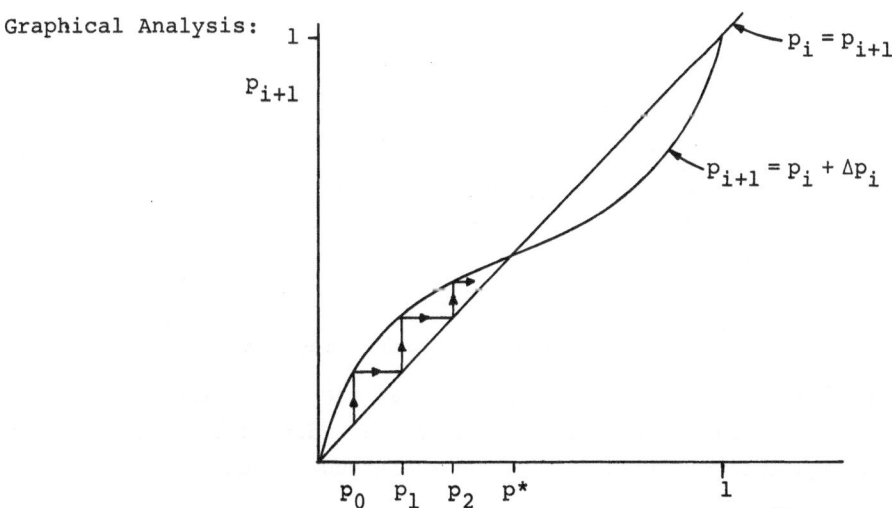

The illustration above represents the case of Heterosis. By projecting first vertically to the curved line and then horizontally to the straight line, sucessive values of p_i can be determined as shown. Note that Heterosis is stable at $(p_i, q_i) = (p*, q*)$.

Sickle Cell Anemia

Sickle cell anemia is actually a combination of cases 1 and 2. In Africa, where malaria is endemic, sickle cell anemia is widespread. The explanation is as follows. There are two alleles, ordinarily called + (normal) and s (sickle). Individuals who are recessive homozygotes die of the disease, but those who are heterozygotes have better resistance to malaria than dominant homozygotes. This leads to the set of fitness relations:

$$W_{++} \; < \; W_{+s} \; > \; W_{ss} \; = \; 0$$

This is of course Heterosis as described above under Case 2. This explains how the s allele found its way into the population.

The descendants of the population with the s allele well established moved to other parts of the world. Many American Blacks can trace their ancestry to the malaria endemic part of Africa. Conditions in this country (where there is no malaria) no longer favor the heterozygotes, so here the fitness relations are:

$$W_{++} \; > \; W_{+s} \; > \; W_{ss} \; = \; 0$$

As described under Case 1, this will lead slowly to the elimination of the s allele by the process of purification.

Problems

1. Given the following data:

$$(D_0, H_0, R_0) \; = \; (1/10, 7/10, 2/10)$$

   a. Find (p_0, q_0)

   b. Find (D_1, H_1, R_1) and (D_2, H_2, R_2)

   c. Plot these results on a De Finetti Diagram.

2. Devise a geometric proof to show that the sum of the perpendicular distances from the three sides to any point within an equilateral triangle with unit altitude is unity.

3. Using any of the expressions from the model with selection,

a. derive the expression:

$$\Delta p_i = p_i q_i (\overline{W}_{i,A} - \overline{W}_{i,a}) / \overline{W}_i$$

b. derive the expression:

$$\Delta p_i = \frac{p_i q_i}{2\overline{W}_i} \frac{d\overline{W}_i}{dp_i}$$

4. Work through the Heterosis case, $W_{AA} < W_{Aa} > W_{aa}$, to show:

a. The location of the equilibrium gene frequency, p*.
b. That p* is a stable equilibrium point, using the analytic method outlined in the section on stability analysis.

5. Repeat the graphical stability analysis performed in the text but for the case of Incompatibility: $W_{AA} > W_{Aa} < W_{aa}$.

References

Models for Hardy-Weinberg Equilibrium and sickle cell anemia can be found in virtually any intermediate level text on genetics. The books noted below are unusually good sources of information:

Bodmer, W.F. and L.L. Cavalli-Sforza, <u>Genetics, Evolution, and Man</u>, W.H. Freeman, San Francisco, 1976.

This is a fascinating and lucid treatment of a difficult subject. The material associated with this section will be found in non-mathematical form in Chapter 9.

Hoppensteadt, F., <u>Mathematical Theories of Populations: Demographics, Genetics, and Epidemics</u>, Society for Industrial and Applied Mathematics, Philadelphia, 1975.

The second section of this short monograph deals with deterministic models in genetics. The continuous time version of the Hardy-Weinberg model is formulated and several special cases are solved. The level of treatment is fairly advanced.

Problem Solutions

Chapter 1: Deterministic Epidemic Models

1. $I(t) = I_o \exp \{ \int_0^t B(\xi)\, d\xi \}$

3. $t_{max} = \frac{1}{N\beta} \ell n \{ (N-I_o)/I_o \}$

    Symmetry — transform origin of independent variable to t_{max}.

4. $R(t) = \frac{\rho I_o}{(S_o-\rho)} [\exp\{\gamma (S_o-\rho)t/\rho\} - 1] \rightarrow \infty$ at $t \rightarrow \infty$ if $S_o > \rho$.

6. By using the third differential equation and then the fact that $S = N - I - R$, one can find $I(t)$ and $S(t)$ without having to solve another differential equation.

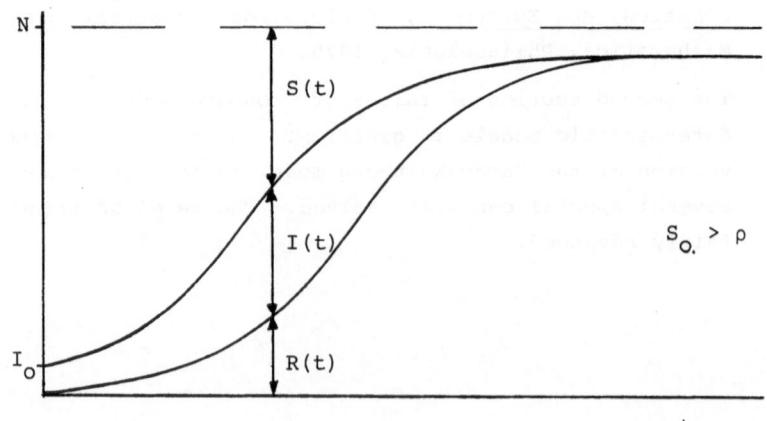

Chapter 2: Rumors and Mousetraps

1. One solution proceeds as follows. Assume that all three types of villages are equally apt to make a call and that the average duration of all calls is τ units of clock time. At model time k there are i_k villages of type I, hence

$$\text{prob \{state-changing call\}} = \frac{i_k}{N+1}$$

   Continue this idea to find the (geometric) probability of j non-state-changing calls prior to a state-changing call, and then find the expectation.

3. $\text{Error} = \dfrac{1 + \lambda \exp\{-\lambda\}}{N} + O(1/N^2)$

5. $I(x) = \exp\{2(k-1)(x-1)/(k-1)\}$

6. Use the differential equation given in problem 5.

Chapter 3: Stochastic Epidemic Models

2. $E[I(t)] = m \exp\{\lambda t\}$
   $V[I(t)] = m \exp\{\lambda t\}[\exp\{\lambda t\} - 1]$

3. $p_3(t) = \exp\{-3\lambda t\} - 2\exp\{-2\lambda t\} + \exp\{-\lambda t\}$

5. $\dfrac{\partial P}{\partial t} = -\lambda s(1-s)\dfrac{\partial P}{\partial s}$
   $p_i(t) = \exp\{-\lambda t\}[1 - \exp\{-\lambda t\}]^{i-1}$

6. Start with the definition

$$E''[I(t)] = \sum_{i=1}^{N} i\, p_i''(t)$$

   and then use the derivative of the Differential-Difference Equation.

Chapter 4: Chain Binomial Models

1. $\sigma_\infty \approx 0.05452$

2. $(s_1, i_1) = (1.5, 1.5)$
   $(s_2, i_2) = (0.530, 0.970)$
   $(s_3, i_3) = (0.271, 0.259)$
   $(s_4, i_4) = (0.226, 0.045)$

3. This problem is long but easy:
   $(E\{s_1\}; E\{I_1\}) = (1.5, 1.5)$
   $(E\{s_2\}; E\{I_2\}) = (0.844, 0.656)$

$$(E\{S_3\}, \ E\{I_3\}) = (0.750, \ 0.094)$$
$$(E\{S_4\}, \ E\{I_4\}) = (0.750, \ 0)$$

4.   Prob$\{0, 1, 2, 3$ removals$\} = (1/8, \ 3/32, \ 3/16, \ 19/32)$

5. $(S_0, \ I_0) = (3, \ 1)$
     $(S_1, \ I_1) = (2, \ 1)$
     $(S_2, \ I_2) = (1, \ 1)$
     $(S_3, \ I_3) = (1, \ 0)$

6.   Same results as in problem 4, but much easier to determine.

Chapter 5: Branching Process Model

2. $f(x) = \dfrac{1}{1 + (1-x) \ \lambda/\mu}$

     $E\{j\} = f'(1) = \lambda/\mu$

4a. $g(y) = \dfrac{\lambda + \mu}{2\lambda} \left[1 - \sqrt{1 - \dfrac{4\lambda\mu y}{(\lambda+\mu)^2}} \ \right]$

4b. $q_1 = \dfrac{\mu}{\lambda + \mu}$

     $q_2 = \dfrac{\lambda\mu^2}{(\lambda + \mu)^3}$

     $q_3 = \dfrac{2\lambda^2\mu^3}{(\lambda + \mu)^5}$

     etc.

5a. $N = 3$

5b. $q_0 = 0, \quad q_1 = 0.60, \quad q_2 = 0.144, \quad q_3 = 0.069$

Chapter 6: Smallpox vaccination discontinuation

5. $\dfrac{d}{dt} P_y = \lambda n (y-1) P_{y-1} - (\lambda n + \mu) y \, P_y + \mu (y+1) P_{y+1}$

7. $s^* = \dfrac{\mu}{\lambda N} [1 - \{\dfrac{365\alpha\lambda\nu}{\omega\beta(1-\ell+\ell/k)}\}^{\frac{1}{2}}]$

Chapter 7: Schistosomiasis Eradication

3.   Consider the region nearer to the origin which looks like the figure below.

     Since the straight line can only be crossed from above and the curved line only from the right, once the region is entered the trajectory must go to the origin.

     An analogous argument applies to the other region.

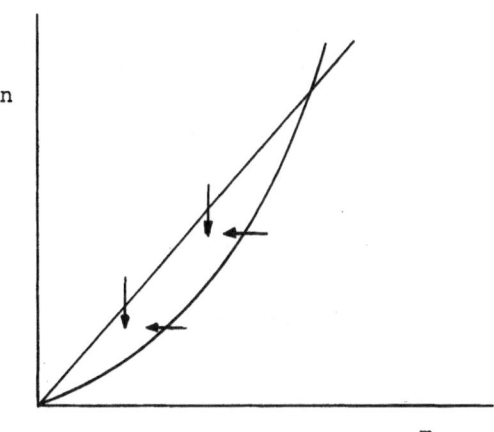

Chapter 8: Gonorrhea

1.   Use a contradiction argument modeled after the one in the chapter.

2.   Parameterize the region as shown below:

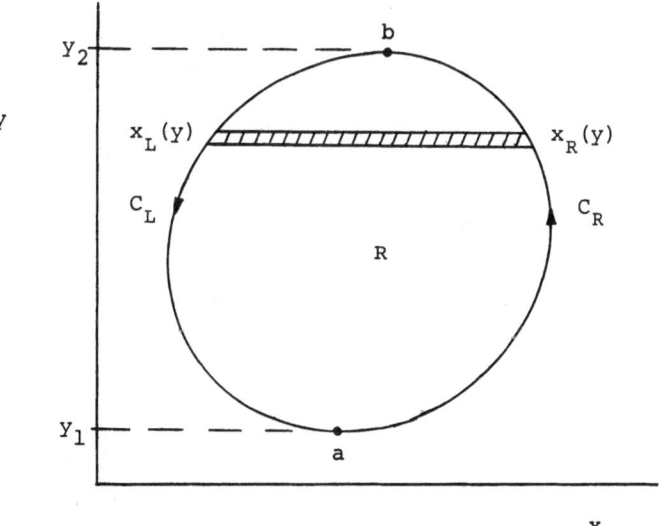

$$\iint_R \frac{\partial U}{\partial x} dx\, dy = \int_{y_1}^{y_2} \int_{x_L(y)}^{x_R(y)} \frac{\partial U}{\partial x} dx\, dy$$

$$= \int_{y_1}^{y_2} U(x_R, y)\, dy - \int_{y_1}^{y_2} U(x_L, y)\, dy$$

$$= \int_{C_R} U(x,y)\, dy + \int_{C_L} U(x,y)\, dy$$

$$= \oint_C U(x,y)\, dy$$

In a similar fashion, it follows that:

$$\iint_R \frac{\partial V}{\partial y}\, dx\, dy = -\oint_C V(x,y)\, dx$$

3. Observe that

$$f(I_1) \;\to\; \begin{cases} 0 & \text{at } I_1 = 0 \\ \infty & \text{as } I_1 \to N_1 \end{cases}$$

$$g(I_1) \;\to\; \begin{cases} 0 & \text{at } I_1 = 0 \\ N_2 & \text{as } I_1 \to \infty \end{cases}$$

$$f'(0) = \frac{\gamma_1}{\beta_1 N_1}, \qquad g'(0) = \frac{\beta_2 N_2}{\gamma_2}$$

3a. If $\beta_1\beta_2 N_1 N_2 > \gamma_1\gamma_2$, $g'(0) > f'(0)$, and the isoclines and arrows look like

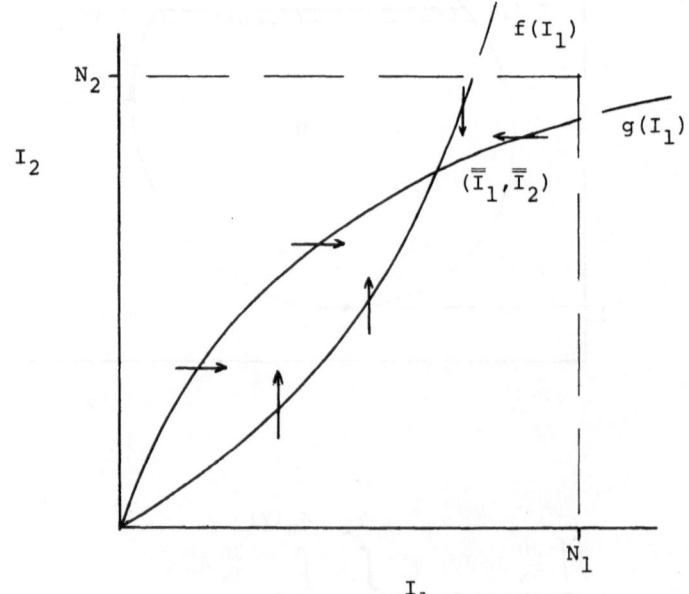

3b. If $\beta_1\beta_2 N_1 N_2 < \gamma_1\gamma_2$, $g'(0) < f'(0)$, and the isoclines and arrows
     look like

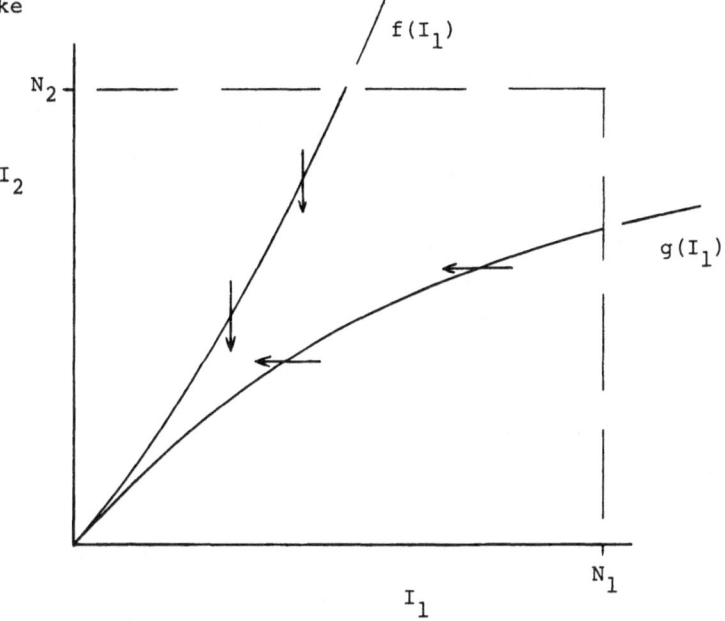

4a. Equilibrium occurs at $I = 0$ and at $I* = N - \frac{\gamma}{\beta}$

4b. Equilibrium point at $I = I*$ is stable when $I* > 0$.

5.   Since $N \to K$ as $t \to \infty$, system moves to $I = 0$ if $K \leq \gamma/\beta$ and to
     $I = K - \gamma/\beta$ if $K > \gamma/\beta$.

Chapter 9: Sickle Cell Anemia

1a. $(p_0, q_0) = (9/20, 11/20)$

1b. $(D_1, H_1, R_1) = (D_2, H_2, R_2) = (81/400, 198/400, 121/400)$

1c.

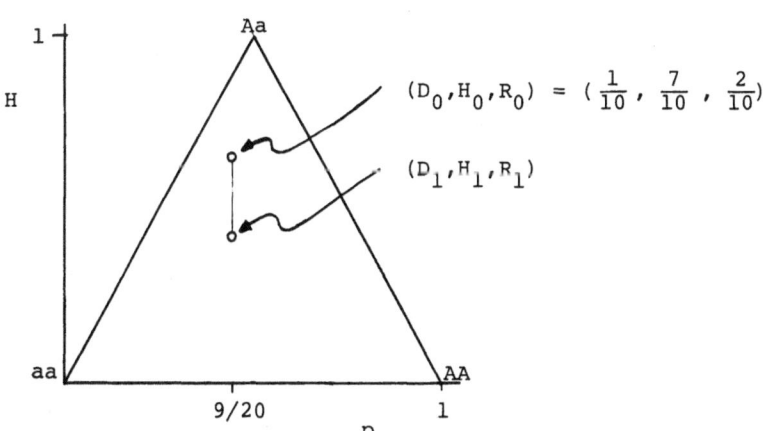

2. Given equilateral triangle with unit altitude:

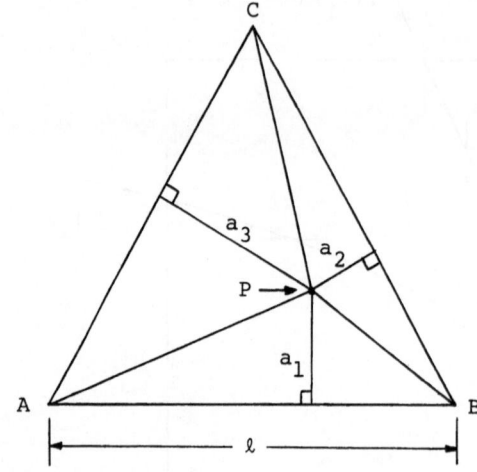

Area (ABC) = $(\ell)(1)$
Area (ABP) = $\ell\, a_1$
Area (BCP) = $\ell\, a_2$
Area (CAP) = $\ell\, a_3$

but Area (ABC) = Area (ABP) + Area (BCP) + Area (CAP)

$$\ell = \ell(a_1 + a_2 + a_3) \quad \rightarrow \quad a_1 + a_2 + a_3 = 1$$

4. $p^* = \dfrac{W_{aa} - W_{Aa}}{W_{AA} - 2W_{Aa} + W_{aa}}$

Subject Index

Bio-mathematics

Managing Editors: K. Krickeberg, S. A. Levin

Volume 8
A. T. Winfree

The Geometry of Biological Time

1980. 290 figures. XIV, 530 pages
ISBN 3-540-09373-7

The widespread appearance of periodic patterns in nature reveals that many living organisms are communities of biological clocks. This landmark text investigates, and explains in mathematical terms, periodic processes in living systems and in their non-living analogues. Its lively presentation (including many drawings), timely perspective and unique bibliography will make it rewarding reading for students and researchers in many disciplines.

Volume 9
W. J. Ewens

Mathematical Population Genetics

1979. 4 figures, 17 tables. XII, 325 pages
ISBN 3-540-09577-2

This graduate level monograph considers the mathematical theory of population genetics, emphasizing aspects relevant to evolutionary studies. It contains a definitive and comprehensive discussion of relevant areas with references to the essential literature. The sound presentation and excellent exposition make this book a standard for population geneticists interested in the mathematical foundations of their subject as well as for mathematicians involved with genetic evolutionary processes.

Volume 10
A. Okubo

Diffusion and Ecological Problems: Mathematical Models

1980. 114 figures, 6 tables. XIII, 254 pages
ISBN 3-540-09620-5

This is the first comprehensive book on mathematical models of diffusion in an ecological context. Directed towards applied mathematicians, physicists and biologists, it gives a sound, biologically oriented treatment of the mathematics and physics of diffusion.

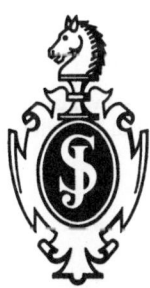

Springer-Verlag
Berlin
Heidelberg
New York

Lecture Notes in Biomathematics

Managing Editor: S. Levin

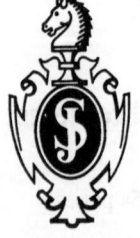

Springer-Verlag
Berlin
Heidelberg
New York

Volume 30
M. Eisen

Mathematical Models in Cell Biology and Cancer Chemotherapy

1979. 70 figures, 17 tables. IX, 431 pages
ISBN 3-540-09709-0

Contents: Introduction. – Cells. – Modelling and Cell Growth. – Some Kinetic Cell Models. – Autoradiography. – Cell Synchrony. – Flow Microfluorometry. – Control Theory. – Towards Mathematical Chemotherapy. – Mathematical Models of Leukopoiesis and Leukemia. – Chemistry of Genes. Protein Synthesis. – Viruses. – Cellular Energy. – Immunology. – Mathematical Theories of Carcinogenesis. – Radiology and Cancer. – Applications of Control Theory to Normal and Malignant Cell Growth. – Index.

Volume 31
E. Akin

The Geometry of Population Genetics

1979. 1 table. IV, 205 pages
ISBN 3-540-09711-2

Contents: Introduction. – The Vectorfield Model of Population Genetics. – The Geometry of Epistasis. – Selection, Recombination and Mutation. – The Hopf Bifurcation. – Appendix. – Bibliography. – Index.

Volume 32

Systems Theory in Immunology

Proceedings of the Working Conference, Held in Rome, May 1978
Editors: C. Bruni, G. Doria, G. Koch, R. Strom

1979. 77 figures, 17 tables. XI, 273 pages
ISBN 3-540-09728-7

Contents: Antigenic Stimulation. – Cell Interactions. – Evaluation and Evolution of Antibody Production. – Mathematical Modeling in Immunology. – The Network Approach.

Volume 33

Mathematical Modelling in Biology and Ecology

Proceedings of a Symposium Held at the CSIR, Pretoria, July 1979
Editor: W. M. Getz

1980. 91 figures, 16 tables. VII, 355 pages
ISBN 3-540-09735-X